Human Well-Being Research a

Series Editors

Richard J. Estes, School of Social Policy & Practice, U͟ ͟ ͟ ͟ ͟ ͟ ͟ ...sylvania,
Philadelphia, PA, USA

M. Joseph Sirgy ⓘ, Department of Marketing, Virginia Polytechnic Institute & State
University, Blacksburg, VA, USA

This series includes policy-focused books on the role of the public and private sectors in advancing quality of life and well-being. It creates a dialogue between well-being scholars and public policy makers. Well-being theory, research and practice are essentially interdisciplinary in nature and embrace contributions from all disciplines within the social sciences. With the exception of leading economists, the policy relevant contributions of social scientists are widely scattered and lack the coherence and integration needed to more effectively inform the actions of policy makers. Contributions in the series focus on one more of the following four aspects of well-being and public policy:

- Discussions of the public policy and well-being focused on particular nations and worldwide regions
- Discussions of the public policy and well-being in specialized sectors of policy making such as health, education, work, social welfare, housing, transportation, use of leisure time
- Discussions of public policy and well-being associated with particular population groups such as women, children and youth, the aged, persons with disabilities and vulnerable populations
- Special topics in well-being and public policy such as technology and well-being, terrorism and well-being, infrastructure and well-being.

This series was initiated, in part, through funds provided by the Halloran Philanthropies of West Conshohocken, Pennsylvania, USA. The commitment of the Halloran Philanthropies is to "inspire, innovate and accelerate sustainable social interventions that promote human well-being." The series editors and Springer acknowledge Harry Halloran, Tony Carr and Audrey Selian for their contributions in helping to make the series a reality.

Jennifer L. Johs-Artisensi • Kevin E. Hansen

Quality of Life and Well-Being for Residents in Long-Term Care Communities

Perspectives on Policies and Practices

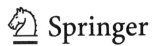

Jennifer L. Johs-Artisensi ⓘ
Department of Management
and Marketing
University of Wisconsin–Eau Claire
Eau Claire, WI, USA

Kevin E. Hansen ⓘ
Department of Health Care Administration
and Public Health
Bellarmine University
Louisville, KY, USA

ISSN 2522-5367   ISSN 2522-5375   (electronic)
Human Well-Being Research and Policy Making
ISBN 978-3-031-04697-1   ISBN 978-3-031-04695-7   (eBook)
https://doi.org/10.1007/978-3-031-04695-7

This Springer imprint is published by the registered company Springer Nature Switzerland AG
The registered company address is: Gewerbestrasse 11, 6330 Cham, Switzerland

I dedicate this book to my family and friends who have supported me throughout the writing process.

My husband, John, has always encouraged my professional pursuits, as he picks up extra responsibilities at home and keeps me caffeinated, fed, and comfortable when I'm writing at nights and on weekends.

As I've worked on this book, my incredible children, Alexis and Evan, have sacrificed time with me, but I hope they have seen that with education, determination, and a strong work ethic, they can do hard things.

I'm so appreciative that my friend Kevin agreed to co-author this book with me—deciding to tackle this together is what made it feel possible.

My other biggest cheerleaders have been my sister, Stephanie, my parents, Carol and Perry, and my friend Lindsey—so thank you for all your words of encouragement along the way.

I fell in love with working with older adults in my 20s and their unique stories changed the trajectory of my career, but one incredible older woman has been an inspiration and role model for my entire life—my grandma Melba. She taught me that a strong, independent woman can do anything, including living her long, final chapter with love, family, meaning, and peace.

Growing older is both a challenge and a privilege. We can all play a role in maximizing older adults' quality of life and well-being as they continue their journey through the life course.
—Jennifer L. Johs-Artisensi

To my work colleagues and friends, my sincere thanks for helping carry the load and for being a constant source of inspiration and wisdom for improving care and quality of life for older adults.

To my friends, too innumerable to list here, thank you for keeping me grounded and for making me take a break now and again for an adult beverage.

To my co-author "Johs," thanks for putting up with me, for our long Zoom calls making each other laugh, and for being a constant cheerleader to work on this book, an undertaking I would not have considered without your willingness to jump in and partner on. We're even, now.

To my dog Thor, destroyer of books and master of sass, we are done with the long weekends in the office, buddy. Thanks for napping and snoring loudly under my desk to keep me company.

Lastly, and most importantly, to my mom Sheri—quite possibly the most amazing social worker and grandma that I know—thank you for listening to me, pushing me to be my best, caring for others as much as you do, and for always being there when you were needed. Love you more than you know, lady.
—Kevin E. Hansen

Acknowledgement

Sadly, after completing final edits on our manuscript, but prior to its publication, Dr. Kevin Hansen unexpectedly passed away, way too soon. His passion for education, research, and elder care rights has already improved care and services for older adults, and he will continue to effect positive change as his knowledge and desire to enhance the lives of older adults is shared through this book. Although he still had so much left to do in this world, his reach will continue, as everyone who knew him carries his influence in their heart.

Author's Note

Jennifer L. Johs-Artisensi, Department of Management and Marketing, University of Wisconsin—Eau Claire, Eau Claire, WI. Kevin E. Hansen, Department of Health and Aging Services Leadership, College of Health Professions, Bellarmine University, Louisville, KY.

The content included in this book has been independently produced by the authors based on their experience, knowledge, and research into existing literature and studies. To date, the authors have received no specific grant, financial support, or reimbursement for the research, authorship, or work toward publication of this submission from any funding agency in the public, commercial, or nonprofit sectors.

Any correspondence concerning this content should be addressed to: Jennifer Johs-Artisensi, Department of Management and Marketing, University of Wisconsin—Eau Claire, 105 Garfield Avenue, Eau Claire, WI 54702.

Email: johsarjl@uwec.edu

Contents

About the Authors

Jennifer Johs-Artisensi is a Professor and Academic Program Director for the Health Care Administration Program at the University of Wisconsin-Eau Claire, and Director of the National Emerging Leadership Summit. She has a master's degree in public health and a PhD in health psychology and behavioral medicine. She has worked as both a practitioner and a consultant in settings across the care continuum. Her research interests include resident-focused care, "culture change" and quality of life in long-term care, health care policy, health and long-term care management, health care administration education, and leadership development. In the USA, she has served the National Association of Long Term Care Administrator Boards (NAB), in multiple capacities, and is the current Chair-Elect of the NAB Executive Committee. She developed an online preceptor training course for NAB, which is used nationwide. She has earned several honors for both her research and service in long-term care, including several Distinguished and Best Paper awards for research on developing educational models to best prepare future long-term care administrators and delivering quality care. She also received the Leon Brachman Award for Community Service, and faculty awards for excellence in service-learning, creativity and innovation, and outstanding teaching.

Kevin Hansen is an Associate Professor and Chair of the Department of Health Care Administration and Public Health at Bellarmine University. His research primarily focuses on quality of care and quality of life in nursing homes, as well as abuse and neglect of vulnerable adults and substitute decision-making with powers of attorney, health care directives, and guardianships and conservatorships. Dr. Hansen has taught courses related to health law and policy, quality improvement in long-term care organizations, leadership in health care settings, ethical and legal issues in aging, elder abuse and neglect, legal issues within health care administration, risk management in health care, and long-term care facility operations. Dr. Hansen has previously taught at the University of Wisconsin-Eau Claire and at the University of South Florida. He has worked as an attorney and ombudsman specialist with the Minnesota Ombudsman Office for Mental Health and Developmental

Disabilities, and as an attorney and victim advocate at the ElderCare Rights Alliance. He has worked in the areas of elder and disability law conducting research and pursuing legislative reform in Minnesota. Dr. Hansen earned his PhD in Aging Studies from the University of South Florida, a Juris Doctor from the William Mitchell College of Law, and a Master of Laws in Elder Law from the Stetson University College of Law.

List of Figures

List of Tables

List of Exhibits

Chapter 1
Quality of Life in Long-Term Care

Quality is the result of a carefully constructed cultural environment. It has to be the fabric of the organization, not part of the fabric. – Phil Crosby

Abstract The population is aging across the globe. Various definitions and over-arching concepts inherent in understanding quality of life for residents in long-term care settings will be introduced to offer readers a common understanding. "Long-term care" will also be defined, as used throughout the book, to include both nursing homes (skilled nursing facilities), assisted living facilities, and other forms of congregate housing with various services provided, along with an examination of factors that may lead to the usage of residential care. The inter-relationship of quality of care and quality of life will be discussed, along with some rationale for its consideration. The current landscape of regulations and policies germane to the provision of high quality of life, including government regulations and implemented policies, will be introduced. The various stakeholders inherent in long-term care communities that have the potential to affect, positively or adversely, resident quality of life will be presented, including front-line and other staff members, leadership (i.e., administration), fellow residents, and family. The content will cover, as an overview, the domain-specific, multifaceted considerations for quality of life that will be addressed in greater detail in subsequent chapters (e.g., dining services, activities, relationships, autonomy, individualized care).

Keywords Older adults · Population aging · Long-term care · Care communities · Assisted living · Nursing homes · Congregate living · Residential care · Person-centered care · Homelike environment · Emotional well-being · Sense of purpose · Hospitality · Culture change · Quality of care · Stakeholders · Quality of life domains

The quality of life for residents in long-term care settings is a multifaceted and complex subject. Quality of life has been researched for many years in efforts to enhance and improve the experience of care recipients in numerous ways. This book introduces and discusses the various definitions, domains, and overarching concepts necessary for administrators, executive directors, and staff members to fully embrace quality of life improvements to enhance resident well-being. While financial considerations and regulatory requirements must be considered, there are myriad changes that can be made within contemporary care centers if the drive and desire exist to enhance resident care. The domains relevant—and covered in this book—to long-term care residents include dining services, activities, relationships, autonomy and respect, environmental surroundings, and individualized care, and care centers have the ability to shape resident experiences in each of these important areas. Throughout this book, examples from congregate long-term care settings primarily seen in Western cultures are shared, yet the tenets described in each domain-specific chapter are applicable to multiple forms of congregate living and cultural practices seen throughout the world.

1.1 Aging Demographics across the Globe

Older adults comprise a large and increasing proportion of the population (Figs. 1.1 and 1.2). In the United States alone there are over 54 million individuals over the age of 65 (U.S. Census Bureau, 2020), and over 700 million worldwide (United Nations,

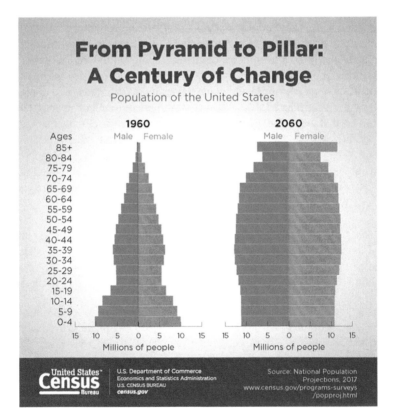

Fig. 1.1 From pyramid to pillar: a century of change (population of the United States). National Population Projections, 2017. United States Census Bureau, Department of Commerce

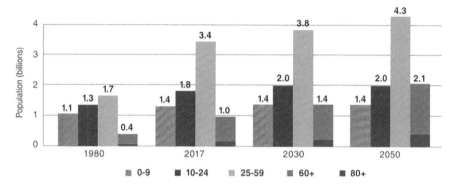

Fig. 1.2 Global Population by Broad Age Group, in 1980, 2017, 2030, and 2050. United Nations, World Population Prospects: The 2017 Revision (2017)

2019), and these numbers are expected to double by 2050 (United Nations, 2020; U.S. Census Bureau, 2014). Studies suggest that the natural aging process, compounded by impacts of disease and disability, will lead to nearly 70% of seniors eventually needing some type of long-term services and supports. Among those who do, the length of service provision will likely last two to four years, with 20% needing care for longer than five years (Administration for Community Living, 2021). Given these vast numbers of people needing long-term services and supports, it is critically important to ensure not only the infrastructure to provide quality clinical care, but that such care is structured with an eye toward maximizing quality of life and resident well-being.

1.2 Defining "Good" Quality of Life

Over time, as the definition of health has evolved away from "the absence of disease" toward a "state of physical, mental, and social well-being" (World Health Organization [WHO], 1946), it became clear that quality of life was a key component of health (Fallowfield, 1990). The WHO defines quality of life as a multi-dimensional, broad concept that includes an individual's subjective evaluation of their physical health, psychological state, independence, social relationships, personal beliefs, and their environment. Many definitions of quality of life have been espoused over the years, oftentimes including elements of enjoyment (Svensson, 1991; Ball et al., 2000), life satisfaction (Ratcliffe et al., 2013; Kelley-Gillespie, 2009), or a sense of meaning or purpose (Johs-Artisensi et al., 2020; Irving et al., 2017; Haugan, 2014; Sarvimaki & Stenbock-Hult, 2000). If anything has become evident in the quality of life literature, it is that quality of life is assessed differently by different people, and its meaning varies across applications (Fayers & Machin, 2016).

Significant research has examined what *good* quality of life means in old age, with Vanleerberghe et al., 2017 concluding that the lack of consensus on a standard definition underscores its subjective nature. Even agreement about the domains of the concept is difficult to come by, although among those who have elaborated on domains contributing to older adults' quality of life, common themes include social, health and physical well-being, and environment (Vanleerberghe et al., 2017), underscoring that quality of life for older adults is a multi-dimensional construct (Schenk et al., 2013). More recently, specific examination of what quality of life means to long-term care recipients has been studied (Johs-Artisensi et al., 2020; Schenk et al., 2013; Shippee et al., 2015; Vaarama, 2009; Degenholtz et al., 2008; Kane 2001, 2003).

1.3   Long-Term Care Communities

As people get older the likelihood they may need long-term care increases, as noted above. Long-term care refers to a wide range of services and supports to help individuals with personal care needs by offering assistance with activities of daily living or other everyday tasks. Depending on the extent of their needs, such care may also involve the provision of supportive medical care. Although many people may be able to receive long-term care services and supports at home either from family or friends or through various community support services, individuals with higher needs may be best served by some type of residential care provider. Residential care includes a variety of assisted living options or, for those with increased care needs, nursing homes may provide the most suitable, comprehensive care.

The term "assisted living" is often used as an umbrella term encompassing providers of board and care, memory care, or other services, whereby recipients leave the home they were previously residing to move into a congregate living setting. In such settings, residents can receive comprehensive services, including lodging, meals, personal care assistance, supervision, socialization, recreational activities, and possibly limited medical assistance—depending on the resident's needs and interests. In contrast, those having higher acuity medical, rehabilitation, behavioral, or psychiatric care needs may be more likely to receive care in more traditional nursing home settings.

Many traditional nursing homes, at their inception, were built around a "medical model" of care, which tended to be more institutional in environmental design. A common physical structure may have been a large building, built of cinderblock walls and tile floors, filled with shared rooms, with multiple long hallways meeting around a large, centralized nurses' station. Operationally, services were often designed primarily around efficiencies for the staff, with pre-scheduled meal times, bedtimes, showers, and activities (Figs. 1.3 and 1.4).

In contrast, over time, there emerged a new type of assisted living provider— constructed around a more social model of care—often with smaller buildings that housed fewer residents and employed a smaller staff who provided a more homelike, physical environment and a culture oriented toward allowing care recipients increased independence and autonomy. Over the past several decades, this

Fig. 1.3 A shared room in Windsor Park Nursing Home, Jamaica, New York. Photo Credit: Gottscho-Schleisner Collection, Library of Congress, Prints and Photographs Division

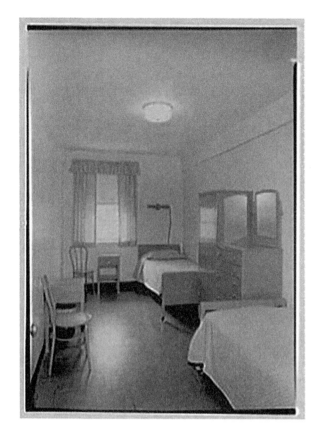

philosophy of more person-centered care has been found to make life better for care recipients and maximize their well-being (Koren, 2010). This approach has since become more widely embraced by all types of long-term care providers (Johs-Artisensi et al., 2021), regardless of the specific care setting (Fig. 1.5).

In this text, all types of congregate living are included—nursing homes, board and care homes, memory care, assisted living, and group homes—any setting in which paid staff are responsible for the provision of long-term services and supports to older adults who live in the same building. For the sake of clarity, the term "long-term care" is broadly used in this book to refer to this constellation of congregate living settings and services provided therein.

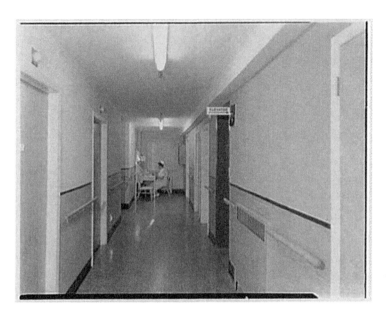

Fig. 1.4 A double loaded corridor leading to the nurse's desk in Windsor Park Nursing Home, Jamaica, New York. Photo Credit: Gottscho-Schleisner Collection, Library of Congress, Prints and Photographs Division

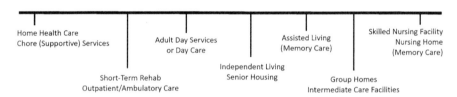

Fig. 1.5 A depiction of the continuum of care of selected long-term service and support settings

1.4 The Decision to Move into a Long-Term Care Community

Every person ages differently, with many facing varied health challenges as time goes by. Sometimes such changes make it more difficult for a person to do and enjoy things that used to come easily. There are many scenarios that may precipitate the decision-making process to move to a supportive residential care environment, like assisted living or a nursing home. A common scenario may include an older adult who has developed multiple medical problems or physical disabilities, and may find themselves needing more day-to-day, hands-on help. Another common situation is when a senior begins to exhibit memory loss, which can be a symptom of Alzheimer's disease or other types of cognitive impairment. Dementia has a tendency to worsen over time, so individuals experiencing it benefit from enhanced supervision, especially if they tend to wander. Often, individuals with dementia may fare well, initially, with support from a spouse, but caregiver burnout is high among those looking after individuals with cognitive impairment. The decision to transition to a memory care center may be the best way to support the individual, while also helping the caregiver to experience a better quality of life, as well. Several signals may indicate such need, as shown in Exhibit 1.1. Finally, another common scenario may include an older adult who has recently lost their spouse. If the spouse was the primary person responsible for tasks such as housework, shopping, and meal preparation, the recently widowed person may find it difficult to learn and carry out such responsibilities in the wake of their loss.

Exhibit 1.1 Signals That a Move to Residential Care May Be in an Individual's Best Interest
- A worsening of medical conditions, an increased number of falls and overall increased frailty.
- Difficulty managing domestic finances or other money problems.
- Difficulty keeping the house clean and a decline in ability to care for oneself.
- Depression or social isolation.

Adapted from U.S. News and World Report's "When to Move From Independent Living to Assisted Living" (Howley, 2019).

Assessing whether such a living transition is the best decision for an individual can be clouded with fears. Change is difficult for everyone, and the fears associated with uprooting one's entire life can feel overwhelming. One of the biggest worries individuals often express is they fear losing their independence—that they will no longer be able to make decisions for themselves and that all their daily actions and routines will be controlled by others. Another common concern is they worry they will be bored and lonely, shut away with nothing to do and no one to visit with them. And when such a change is being contemplated in the wake of the loss of a partner or one's own losses associated with physical or cognitive decline, those fears can be amplified. When spouses or other family members are participating in the decision-making process with the individual who needs care, feelings of guilt may also be a factor. Families may feel they are letting their loved one down if they are no longer able to sustain a primary caregiver role, and families may worry that older loved ones will perceive they have been a burden to the family members providing necessary care. Although the decision to transition to residential care can be a difficult one for individuals and their families to make, in many cases it is the best choice. Both care recipients and their loved ones will feel better about the decision if the individual's new home prioritizes resident quality of life and emotional well-being while simultaneously ensuring high quality of care. Savvy providers recognize that the most common fears of prospective residents relate to the transition and its potential effects on the person's quality of life and emotional well-being. Knowing this, some providers have demonstrated the ability to structure their long-term living environments so that quality of life is a key driver of their model of care and resident satisfaction is an authentic priority in their operations and strategy.

1.5   Influence of Quality of Life on Other Metrics

Quality of life has significant impact on resident satisfaction in long-term care and having "meaning" is crucial for resident satisfaction (Burack et al., 2012). Research suggests that meaning is essential to care recipients' functional and emotional well-being (Haugan, 2014) and is a central component of quality of life (Sarvimaki & Stenbock-Hult, 2000). Additionally, experiencing a higher sense of purpose is correlated with better health and well-being outcomes for older adults (Irving et al., 2017). Thus, recognition of factors that contribute to care recipients' quality of life should be of critical importance to providers of such services and supports.

With evidence that supports the importance of quality of life, not just on well-being but, in turn, its association with positive health outcomes (Centers for Disease Control and Prevention, 2018), long-term care providers are compelled to facilitate both quality care and quality of life as a moral imperative as well as a function of regulatory requirements (Degenholtz et al., 2014). Across North America, Europe, and Asia, governments play a vested role in regulating quality care in congregate settings (Mor et al., 2014), with increasing attention paid to quality of life in recent years (WeDO, 2012). For example, in the United States, policy implications for nursing home resident quality of life emerged following the federal 1987 Omnibus Budget Reconciliation Act (OBRA), more commonly referred to as the Nursing Home Reform Act (42 CFR § 483.24), where providers were required to include specific emphases on activities programming or they would be subject to citations and penalties (Kane et al., 2000). When nursing home regulations were revised in 2017, an even greater emphasis was placed on resident experiences, with requirements for provision of person-centered care and facilitating the highest practicable resident quality of life. Even the process of assessing the impact of such practices was adjusted, placing increased importance on direct resident feedback about their experience living in the facility (Centers for Medicare and Medicaid Services [CMS], 2019).

1.6   Enhancing Resident Quality of Life

Given the importance of resident quality of life on multiple facets of residential care, including the important health and emotional benefits when residents have a good quality of life and the importance of avoiding regulatory penalties, ensuring providers understand how to facilitate care recipient well-being is critical. And beyond regulatory requirements or a moral imperative, it is simply good business. As care providers find themselves in an increasingly competitive market for prospective residents, developing services designed to enhance quality of life and well-being of older adults makes good business sense and may help them distinguish themselves from competitors. Several ideas of low- or no-cost ideas to improve quality of life are shown in Exhibit 1.2. When providers specifically understand their care recipients' lived experiences, they can best meet their needs. Since quality of life is associated with life satisfaction (Ratcliffe et al., 2013; Kelley-Gillespie, 2009), it stands to reason that more satisfied care recipients may more frequently recommend their care communities to others (Berkman & Gilson, 1986). It is known that customer recommendations influence consumers' purchasing decisions (Palmer et al., 2011) and are an economical means of promotion (Knudson, 1988; Naumann, 1995). Thus, senior care providers can and should increase their focus on hospitality and other approaches for improving resident well-being. In turn, they may find that such strategies are also effective methods of increasing their census and prospective revenue sources.

Exhibit 1.2 Advancing Culture Change to Improve Quality of Life Doesn't Have to Cost Anything

Routines for Residents

- Letting residents choose when they'd like to go to bed and when to wake up.
- Work with the medical team to have medications administered at times convenient for the resident.
- Utilize consistent staff assignment practices to develop relationships and gain better familiarity with resident preferences and needs.

Tailoring Care Plans to Residents

- Upon admission to a care center, use an assessment strategy that welcomes the resident and gathers important life information.
- Assure that residents are invited to and actively participate in their care planning sessions, to the degree they wish to be involved and in a location that may encourage participation.

New Employee Hiring Practices and Training

- Incorporate residents into the interview processes for staff.
- As part of onboarding and initial training, having a panel of residents sharing their views on quality of life and quality care can help new staff understand their role.

Resident and Family Councils

(continued)

Exhibit 1.2 (continued)
- Care centers can have a team that meets regularly to discuss culture change and can incorporate representatives from councils to serve on that with staff members.
- A "Welcome Committee" could be created with staff and resident representatives from the council to help a new resident better acclimate to their new home.
- Have tours of the care center include a meeting with representatives from both councils to hear their feedback.

Creating a Sense of Home in the Environment

- Have residents decorate their bedrooms with wall hangings, furniture, and other decorative items.
- Work with residents to create names of neighborhoods in the care center that have meaning to them.
- Have food stations and snack areas scattered throughout the building to promote socialization and food consumption.

Adapted from the National Consumer Voice's "10 No-Cost Ideas to Advance Your Culture Change Journey by Involving Residents and Families" (National Consumer Voice, 2011).

In long-term care, the term "culture change" refers to a foundational shift in the philosophy of how care should be provided in nursing homes and, by extension, other long-term care settings. The main premise of this approach is to allow residents to direct their own care in a more homelike atmosphere where relationships are fostered, staff are empowered to tailor care and services to resident needs, care community decisions are made collaboratively, and quality improvement processes are ongoing. Despite common awareness of these care philosophies and research suggesting these practices improve resident well-being and organizational performance, significant widespread adoption of such practices and approaches to care remains modest (Koren, 2010).

1.7   Quality of Care Vs. Quality of Life

As noted by Castle and Ferguson (2010), "numerous definitions of quality exist." Many studies utilize proxy measures for quality as an intangible goal that cannot be directly measured, referred to in US nursing homes as quality indicators (Castle & Ferguson, 2010; Zimmerman, 2003). A sample of such quality measures can be found in Exhibit 1.3. At the overall facility level, annual re-certification surveys—designed to ensure ongoing compliance with minimal standards of quality set by the

Centers for Medicare and Medicaid Services (CMS)—and the citations for deficient conduct have been used to measure quality within a given nursing home (Castle et al., 2010). Other studies have analyzed quality in terms of complaints related to quality of care, which can emanate from multiple sources and may be investigated separately (Hansen et al., 2019; Stevenson, 2006). Additionally, nurse and nurse aide staffing levels have also been used as a metric of quality (Hyer et al., 2011; Rantz et al., 2004; Shin & Hyun, 2015) as has payer mix (e.g., higher percentages of resident care reimbursed through Medicaid has indicated lower quality of care) (Mor et al., 2004). While many metrics exist to evaluate nursing home quality (e.g., Care Compare; CMS, 2021), fewer public-facing measures are available for assisted living facilities in the United States, for example, given the lack of nationwide standardized surveys, quality of care metrics, and consistent data available for analyses.

Exhibit 1.3 Sample of Quality Measures for Long-Stay Residents in the United States
- Number of hospitalizations per 1000 long-stay resident days.
- Number of outpatient emergency department visits per 1000 long-stay resident days.
- Percent of residents who received an antipsychotic medication.
- Percent of residents experiencing one or more falls with major injury.
- Percent of high-risk residents with pressure ulcers.
- Percent of residents with a urinary tract infection (UTI).
- Percent of residents who have or had a catheter inserted and left in their bladder.
- Percent of residents whose need for help with activities of daily living (ADLs) increased.
- Percent of residents who were physically restrained.
- Percent of low-risk residents who lose control of their bowels or bladder.
- Percent of residents who lose too much weight.
- Percent of residents who have symptoms of depression.
- Percent of residents who used antianxiety or hypnotic medications.

Adapted from the Centers for Medicare and Medicaid Services Long Stay Quality Measures (CMS, 2021).

Beyond facility-level quality indicators, quality of care is also assessed at the resident level or from the residents' perspective (Pearson et al., 1993). While many studies distinguish quality of care from quality of life indicators, others have analyzed the intersectionality of these two concepts. Grabowski et al. (2014) evaluated the impact of culture change programs, typically designed to improve resident quality of life (Koren, 2010), and their effects on the quality of care in a given facility. Some studies even have assessed the impact of quality of care and quality of life near the end of a resident's life, where quality may matter even more (Tilden et al., 2002).

1.8   Balance between Safety and Autonomy

With the attention and emphasis often given to quality of care, quality of life is sometimes overlooked, which is a mistake. While often the provision of quality care supports quality of life, occasionally too much emphasis—especially on certain safety aspects of quality of care—has the potential to hinder quality of life. Conversely, decision-making with consideration of quality of life factors may even have the added benefit of positively influencing quality care. In most countries, one impetus for establishing rules and regulations for long-term care was the public protection of vulnerable adults' safety (Kaiser Family Foundation, 2015). Thus, an underlying thread among many regulations is an emphasis on protecting resident's safety. Although certainly important and well-intentioned, the protection of resident safety often historically has not come without sacrifice, usually at the expense of residents' privacy and autonomy, which are important factors in quality of life. A good example is mitigation of falls risk. Luckily, many care centers have moved away from the obviously restrictive use of restraints. An example of this is provided in Exhibit 1.4. However, it is sometimes still difficult for providers to navigate the balance of affording residents the choice to leave the building, or make other autonomous decisions for themselves (e.g., engaging in preferred activities, eating certain foods which might be deemed "unsafe" for them), which may have significant benefits in sustaining or enhancing the individual's quality of life.

> **Exhibit 1.4 Balancing Safety and Autonomy: A Win–Win**
> After Mrs. Jones sustained several falls at her new nursing facility, she was deemed a "falls risk" and staff began to use a "lap tray", which was effectively a physical restraint to prevent her from getting out of her chair. She was very aware that her bodily autonomy was being restricted and this agitated her, further prompting her to try to get out of the chair and led to significant emotional distress. Her care center was launching a new "no restraints" policy to get into compliance with regulations that required a reduction of restraint use. Staff were worried they were going to see an increase in resident falls without restraints. However, they followed protocols to assess the root causes of Mrs. Jones' previous falls and put a care plan in place incorporating information from several of her daily caregivers who were familiar with her routines. The care plan included additional supervision later in the day, when she tended to be weaker, and for certain activities that were higher risk. They also got her engaged in more social activities to reduce boredom and isolation

(continued)

Exhibit 1.4 (continued)
(which tended to be a trigger for agitation), provided Mrs. Jones with education and instruction on the benefits preventing falls offers her, along with some specific strategies she could use to minimize her own risks, including calling for help prior to attempting self-transfers. Finally, they added additional adaptive equipment in her bathrooms to provide a safer environment.In the first two months after rolling out the new restraint-free care plan, Mrs. Jones and her whole care team were pleasantly surprised to see that not only had she not sustained any new falls, but she was rarely agitated and her emotional distress was significantly reduced. Her mood was elevated, she was much more engaged in activities, and she had made some new friends. Her quality of life was greatly improved. Mrs. Jones' care is an excellent example of how making quality of care decisions in parallel with consideration of quality of life actually led to an improvement of both.

Inherent in allowing residents more autonomy is an element of risk, and the fluid tension between safety and autonomy is real. However, to *completely* mitigate risk will interfere with nearly all elements of what is important to residents' quality of life, significantly reducing their emotional well-being. Instead, a balance must be achieved. When protection of safety is the primary goal, autonomy and other elements of quality of life could be completely forgone, so perhaps maximizing safety is the wrong orientation. In contrast, when maximizing resident quality of life is the driving impetus, by definition, a consideration of safety *must* be part of the equation, and when safety is considered in conjunction with quality of life, it ideally leads to better outcomes for both.

1.9   Resident-Defined Quality of Life

Individuals derive their own sense of meaning for themselves (Drageset et al., 2017); however, if those who design and deliver residential care services have an increased understanding of factors contributing to resident meaning and quality of life, they can facilitate resident experiences and perceptions of these phenomena. Enhanced understanding of how residents themselves define, value, and experience factors related to quality of life supports providers in developing systems, operationalizing practices, and embodying leadership styles to best cultivate person-centered care cultures that emphasize resident quality of life (Johs-Artisensi, 2017).

Among long-term care recipients, there is the very real possibility that some residents are unable to speak for themselves, due to cognitive impairment or physical disability. Because of this, care providers often rely on proxies to speak on residents' behalf but, in resident quality of life research, resident and proxy assessments are often found to be misaligned (Godin et al., 2015; Gerritsen et al., 2007; Kane et al.,

2005) and the components of quality of life that various stakeholders identify as important to care recipients often differ (Johs-Artisensi et al., 2020; Kehyayan et al., 2015; Kane et al., 1997, 2003, 2005). Table 1.1 presents various stakeholder perspectives on contributory factors to resident quality of life and sense of purpose.

Since provider perceptions of resident quality of life cannot reliably replace residents' own perspectives for subjective experiences (Johs-Artisensi et al., 2020; Kane et al., 2005; Andresen et al., 2001), the content in this book attempts to highlight and focus on residents' input and perceptions of quality, providing more accurate information to improve quality of life in long-term care communities.

There are many different stakeholders invested in the provision and quality of care beyond long-term care recipients themselves. Family members, such as a spouse, adult children, or other friends and family, are often motivated to ensure their loved one is receiving quality care and having the best possible quality of life, despite needing care and assistance. Additionally, there are many individuals involved in the provision of said care, including front-line caregivers (e.g., nurses, nurse aides, personal care workers) or even dietary or nutrition aides, housekeepers, or maintenance workers. These staff are augmented by the management team, such as nurse managers, social workers, activities directors, chaplains, and facility administrators, directors, or owners, who are also entrusted with ensuring the care and well-being of care recipients. In Johs-Artisensi et al. (2020), although those in nursing home leadership roles purportedly had care recipients' best interests in mind, there was found to be a meaningful lack of alignment between what administrators, social workers, and activities directors thought were key contributory factors to resident quality of life compared to what residents themselves reported. Compared to management, nursing assistants (i.e., those providing most of the hands-on caregiving) were not entirely attuned with care recipients, but they seemed to have perspectives on contributory factors to resident quality of life that most closely aligned with residents' own perspectives. Subsequent content in this book focuses on the domains which influence quality of life, and key stakeholder roles are highlighted to demonstrate their direct influence within each domain.

1.10   Quality of Life Domains

Chapter 2 lays a foundation for the essential treatment of care recipients as individuals. From a moral imperative to the regulations governing the operations of long-term care facilities, there are specific provisions related to resident dignity, autonomy and choice, respect, privacy (when and to the extent possible), and individualization of the care and services provided, each of which will be covered in turn. As part of resident autonomy, this chapter covers resident councils, as well as the many ways in which facility staff and leadership can and must engage with residents to support them in directing their own care, thereby maximizing resident quality of life. Additionally, research exploring residents' sense of purpose and how long-term care facilities can enhance residents' feelings of self-worth and usefulness in

Table 1.1 Frequency of perceived contributory factors to resident quality of life and sense of purpose

Resident Quality of Life

Stakeholders	First	Second	Third	Fourth	Fifth
Residents	Staff and Resident Relationships	Autonomy and Respect	Sense of Community	Food and Drink	Activities
Nursing Assistants	Staff and Resident Relationships	Autonomy and Respect	Quality of Care	Activities	Food and drink
Activities Directors	Activities	Staff and Resident Relationships	Autonomy and Respect	Quality of Care	Comfortability and environment
Social Workers	Quality of Care	Staff and Resident Relationships	Autonomy and Respect	Activities	Comfortability and environment
Administrators	Staff and Resident Relationships	Quality of Care	Autonomy and Respect	Activities	Comfortability and environment

Resident Sense of Purpose

Stakeholders	First	Second	Third	Fourth	Fifth
Residents	Sense of Community	Activities	Familial Communication	Contributory Service to the Community	Quality of Care
Nursing Assistants	Activities	Autonomy and Respect	Sense of Community and Quality of Care[a]		Staff and Resident Relationships
Activities Directors	Activities	Sense of Community	Autonomy and Respect	Staff and Resident Relationships	Contributory Service to the Community
Social Workers	Activities	Autonomy and Respect	Sense of Community	Quality of Care	Contributory Service to the Community
Administrators	Activities and Sense of Community[b]		Autonomy and Respect	Quality of Care	Contributory Service to the Community

[a]For Nursing Assistants, Sense of Community and Quality of Care had equal frequencies
[b]For Administrators, Activities and Sense of Community had equal frequencies
Adapted from "Qualitative and Quantitative Analysis of Quality of Life Survey Results Research Report" (Hansen et al., 2018)

congregate living settings is examined. Methods to promote a sense of purpose will be addressed, which helps residents experience meaning and improves overall satisfaction and quality of life in long-term care.

Chapter 3 focuses on relationships which substantially impact resident quality of life. Research has indicated that residents value relationships with multiple constituencies. Resident-resident (peer) relationships, resident-staff relationships, and resident-family relationships are all explored. The value of peer relationships and how they contribute to a sense of belonging are examined, including resident preferences for and types of relationships, how proximity and peer activities or engagement opportunities help form such relationships, and how facilities can remove barriers and support residents' relationships with each other. Additionally, interpersonal relationships, including intimate or romantic interactions, that are either pre-established or newly formed after arrival at the care community, will be included. The importance of relationships between staff and residents is also described. Direct care staff often have the greatest potential to affect resident quality of life and, when residents cannot speak for themselves, may serve as accurate proxies for resident preferences. How these relationships support individualized care and emotional well-being is detailed, along with specific approaches and actions to promote such relationships. Finally, the promotion and facilitation of family member visits will be discussed, including options to do so virtually via technology when in-person visits are not feasible. Strategies for building connections with families are also highlighted, including the value of effective family councils.

The content in Chap. 4 focuses on many of the psychosocial aspects that impact resident quality of life in long-term care settings. The number and variety of activities and programs scheduled for long-term care residents serve many purposes: physical activity, socialization, cognitive stimulation, community-building, and more. Intrafacility activities and programs, as well as programming that incorporates external events, stakeholders, and organizations to engage residents with their surrounding community members are addressed. Activities designed or adapted for residents with cognitive impairments and for residents with physical impairments (e.g., residents who are ventilator-dependent) are also covered. Lastly, the religious preferences and practices of residents in long-term care settings are addressed, including informal activities that may be scheduled as well as more formal religious services.

The physical environment influences quality of life for residents in long-term care, especially as it impedes or supports privacy and autonomy, and can particularly affect residents with dementia. The impact of the built environment and evidence-based design practices are explored in Chap. 5, including physical design and re-design of rooms and communal spaces within facilities to promote a homelike environment. This can include the use of smaller spaces, as well as color and design strategies, to maximize resident independence and autonomy. Other content addresses residents' ability to personalize both their own living spaces and to have input into the communal spaces of their home. Additionally, strategic placement of seating options to facilitate socialization and physical activity are addressed, along with examining the value of outside spaces to support well-being and sensory engagement. Lastly, environmental recommendations to support residents with cognitive impairments are made, including environmental cueing, prevention of elopement, and activity stations to alleviate distress and promote engagement.

When interviewing long-term care residents on aspects of their daily lives that have the greatest impact, food—and dining services, overall—often ranks at the very top of the list. Chap. 6 discusses food preparation, dining preferences, selection at meal times, the dining experience, and delivery of meals in long-term care settings. The importance of nutrition and hydration for older adults, as part of carefully crafted menus and meals, is also covered. Attention is paid to distinguishing current approaches in culinary services from more resident-focused, resident-driven best practices (e.g., aligning with culture change principles for individualization). In addition to the selection of dietary items, the setting in which meals are served (e.g., shifts away from gargantuan dining halls to a more restaurant-styled atmosphere) is discussed, as well as different hospitality-centered nomenclature for staff (e.g., "servers" rather than the traditional "dietary aide"). Resident choice and autonomy, including meal preferences, are a focus of this domain that substantially affects quality of life.

In Chap. 7, the medical aspects of care provided in long-term care settings are emphasized. Some of the existing literature distinguishes quality of care from quality of life, while other research explores the interrelated nature of the two concepts. This relationship is explored in depth, emphasizing the individualized medical care (e.g., nursing, specialty care and services, physical therapy, occupational therapy) aspects provided to residents and how care can impact quality of life, including the CMS-enumerated quality measures for short-stay and long-stay residents. The care planning processes and incorporation of residents, residents' family members, or residents' proxy decision-makers in the process are emphasized, as are the inclusion of unique resident-driven preferences and needs to tailor care plans appropriately. Finally, the importance of transitions (i.e., transfers) between various care settings is addressed (e.g., hospital discharge to nursing home for therapy), as poorly executed transfers have negative implications on resident health and quality of life (e.g., transfer trauma, increased cognitive decline, disorientation).

Lastly, while some best practices and brief policy analysis will be included in each of the domain-specific chapters, Chap. 8 will conclude by delving deeper into suggested organizational leadership strategies that administrators and executive directors can employ, as well as macro-level policies designed to focus on the resident and enhance quality of life in care communities. Using existing research and currently implemented practices as a foundation, policy recommendations strive to incorporate current governmental regulations and reimbursement methodologies to enhance the resident experience. While the proposed policy suggestions will center around the domains presented in the book, they will also incorporate the various stakeholder groups, as applicable, and provide practical implementation strategies. Finally, content will focus on conclusions that ultimately augment the planning and delivery of care and services in multiple long-term care settings to enhance quality of life for all residents.

References

Administration for Community Living, United States Department of Health and Human Services. (2021). *How much care will you need?* Retrieved from https://acl.gov/ltc/basic-needs/how-much-care-will-you-need.

Andresen, E. M., Vahle, V. J., & Lollar, D. (2001). Proxy reliability: Health-related quality of life (HRQoL) measures for people with disability. *Quality of Life Research, 10*(7), 609–619.

Ball, M. M., Whittington, F. J., Perkins, M. M., Patterson, V. L., Hollingsworth, C., Sharon, V. K., & Combs, B. L. (2000). Quality of life in assisted living facilities: Viewpoints of residents. *Journal of Applied Gerontology, 19*(3), 304–325. https://doi.org/10.1177/073346480001900304

Berkman, H. W., & Gilson, C. (1986). *Consumer behavior: Concepts and strategies.* Kent Publishing.

Burack, O. R., Weiner, A. S., Reinhardt, J. P., & Annunziato, R. A. (2012). What matters most to nursing home elders: Quality of life in the nursing home. *Journal of the American Medical Directors Association, 13*(1), 48–53. https://doi.org/10.1016/j.jamda.2010.08.002

Castle, N. G., & Ferguson, J. C. (2010). What is nursing home quality and how is it measured? *The Gerontologist, 50*(4), 426–442. https://doi.org/10.1093/geront/gnq052

Castle, N. G., Wagner, L. M., Ferguson, J. C., & Handler, S. M. (2010). Nursing home deficiency citations for safety. *Journal of Aging and Social Policy, 23*(1), 34–57. https://doi.org/10.1080/08959420.2011.532011

Centers for Disease Control and Prevention, United States Department of Health and Human Services. (2018). *Well-being concepts.* Retrieved from https://www.cdc.gov/hrqol/wellbeing.htm#:~:text=Well%2Dbeing%20is%20associated%20with%20numerous%20health%2D%2C%20job%2D,%2C%20and%20economically%2Drelated%20benefits.&text=For%20example%2C%20higher%20levels%20of,speedier%20recovery%3B%20and%20increased%20longevity

Centers for Medicare and Medicaid Services, United States Department of Health and Hman Services. (2021). *Quality measures.* Retrieved from https://www.cms.gov/Medicare/Quality-Initiatives-Patient-Assessment-Instruments/NursingHomeQualityInits/NHQIQualityMeasures

Centers for Medicare and Medicaid Services, United States Department of Health and Human Services. (2019). *Long-term care survey process procedure guide.* Retrieved from https://www.cms.gov/Medicare/Provider-Enrollment-and-Certification/GuidanceforLawsAndRegulations/Downloads/LTCSP-Procedure-Guide.pdf.

Centers for Medicare and Medicaid Services, United States Department of Health and Human Services. (2021). *Care compare.* Retrieved from https://www.medicare.gov/care-compare/

Degenholtz, H. B., Resnick, A. L., Bulger, N., & Chia, L. (2014). Improving quality of life in nursing homes: The structured resident interview approach. *Journal of Aging Research, 2014*, 892679. https://doi.org/10.1155/2014/892679

Degenholtz, H. B., Rosen, J., Castle, N., Mittal, V., & Liu, D. (2008). The association between changes in health status and nursing home resident quality of life. *The Gerontologist, 48*(5), 584–592. https://doi.org/10.1093/geront/48.5.584

Drageset, J., Haugan, G., & Tranvag, O. (2017). Crucial aspects promoting meaning and purpose in life: Perceptions of nursing home residents. *BMC Geriatrics, 17*(1), 1–9. https://doi.org/10.1186/s12877-017-0650-x

Fallowfield, L. (1990). *The quality of life: The missing measurement in health care.* Souvenir Press.

Fayers, P., & Machin, D. (2016). *Quality of life: The assessment, analysis and reporting of patient-reported outcomes.* Wiley-Blackwell.

Gerritsen, D. L., Steverink, N., Ooms, M. E., de Vet, H. C. W., & Ribbe, M. W. (2007). Measurement of overall quality of life in nursing homes through self report: The role of cognitive impairment. *Quality of Life Research, 16*(6), 1029–1037. https://doi.org/10.1007/s11136-007-9203-7

Godin, J., Keefe, J., Kelloway, E. K., & Hirdes, J. P. (2015). Nursing home resident quality of life: Testing for measurement equivalence across resident, family, and staff perspectives. *Quality of Life Research, 24*(10), 2365–2374. https://doi.org/10.1007/s11136-015-0989-4

Grabowski, D. C., O'Malley, A. J., Afendulis, C. C., Caudry, D. J., Elliot, A., & Zimmerman, S. (2014). Culture change and nursing home quality of care. *The Gerontologist, 42*(Suppl. 1), S35–S45. https://doi.org/10.1093/geront/gnt143

Hansen, K. E., Hyer, K., Holup, A. A., Smith, K. M., & Small, B. J. (2019). Analyses of complaints, investigations of allegations, and deficiency citations in United States nursing homes. *Medical Care Research and Review, 76*(6), 736–757. https://doi.org/10.1177/1077558717744863

Hansen, K. E., Johs-Artisensi, J. L., Olson, D., Berg, N., & Parker, K. (2018). *Qualitative and quantitative analysis of quality of life survey results research report.* Center for Health Administration and Aging Services Excellence.

Haugan, G. (2014). Meaning-in-life in nursing-home patients: A correlate with physical and emotional symptoms. *Journal of Clinical Nursing, 23*(7–8), 1030–1043. https://doi.org/10.1111/jocn.12282

Howley, E. K. (2019, August 9). *When to move from independent living to assisted living.* U.S. News and World Report. Retrieved from https://health.usnews.com/best-assisted-living/articles/when-to-move-from-independent-living-to-assisted-living.

Hyer, K., Thomas, K. S., Branch, L. G., Harman, J. S., Johnson, C. E., & Weech-Maldonado, R. (2011). The influence of nurse staffing levels on quality of care in nursing homes. *The Gerontologist, 51*(5), 610–616. https://doi.org/10.1093/geront/gnr050

Irving, J., Davis, S., & Collier, A. (2017). Aging with purpose: Systematic search and review of literature pertaining to older adults and purpose. *International Journal of Aging and Human Development, 85*(4), 403–437. https://doi.org/10.1177/0091415017702908

Johs-Artisensi, J. L. (2017). Operationalizing person-centered care practices in long-term care: Recommendations from a "resident for a day" experience. *Patient Experience Journal, 4*(3), 76–85. https://doi.org/10.35680/2372-0247.1174

Johs-Artisensi, J. L., Hansen, K. E., & Olson, D. M. (2020). Qualitative analyses of nursing home residents' quality of life from multiple stakeholders' perspectives. *Quality of Life Research, 29,* 1229–1238. https://doi.org/10.1007/s11136-019-02395-3

Johs-Artisensi, J. L., Hansen, K. E., Olson, D. M., & Creapeau, L. J. (2021). Leadership perceptions and practices of hospitality in senior care. *Journal of Applied Gerontology, 40*(6), 598–608. https://doi.org/10.1177/0733464820923903

Kaiser Family Foundation. (2015, August 31). *Long-term care in the United States: A timeline.* Retrieved from https://www.kff.org/medicaid/timeline/long-term-care-in-the-united-states-a-timeline/.

Kane, R. A. (2001). Long-term care and a good quality of life: Bringing them closer together. *The Gerontologist, 41*(3), 293–304. https://doi.org/10.1093/geront/41.3.293

Kane, R. A., Caplan, A. L., Urv-Wong, E. K., Freeman, I. C., Aroskar, M. A., & Finch, M. (1997). Everyday matters in the lives of nursing home residents: Wish for and perception of choice and control. *Journal of the American Geriatrics Society, 45*(9), 1086–1093.

Kane, R. L., Kane, R. A., Bershadsky, B., Degenholtz, H., Kling, K., Totten, A., et al. (2005). Proxy sources for information on nursing home residents' quality of life. *Journals of Gerontology, Series B: Psychological Sciences and Social Sciences, 60*(6), S318–S325. https://doi.org/10.1093/geronb/60.6.s318

Kane, R. A., Kane, R. L., Giles, K., Lawton, M. P., Bershadsky, B., & Kling, K. (2000). *First findings from wave 1 data collection: Measures, indicators, and improvement of quality of life in nursing homes.* University of Minnesota, Division of Health Services Research, Policy, and Administration.

Kane, R. A., Kling, K. C., Bershadsky, B., Kane, R. L., Giles, K., Degenholtz, H. B., et al. (2003). Quality of life measures for nursing home residents. *Journals of Gerontology, Series A: Biological Sciences and Medical Sciences, 58*(3), 240–248. https://doi.org/10.1093/gerona/58.3.m240

Kane, R. L., Rockwood, T., Hyer, K., Desjardins, K., Brassard, A., Gessert, C., et al. (2005). Rating the importance of nursing home residents' quality of life. *Journal of the American Geriatrics Society, 53*(12), 2076–2082. https://doi.org/10.1111/j.1532-5415.2005.00493.x

Kehyayan, V., Hirdes, J. P., Tyas, S. L., & Stolee, P. (2015). Residents' self-reported quality of life in long-term care facilities in Canada. *Canadian Journal on Aging, 34*(2), 149–164. https://doi.org/10.1017/S0714980814000579

Kelley-Gillespie, N. (2009). An integrated conceptual model of quality of life for older adults based on a synthesis of the liter-ature. *Applied Research in Quality of Life, 4*(3), 259–282. https://doi.org/10.1007/s11482-009-9075-9

Knudson, B. J. (1988). Ten laws of customer satisfaction. *Cornell Hotel and Restaurant Quarterly, 29*(3), 14–17.

Koren, M. J. (2010). Person-centered care for nursing home residents: The culture-change movement. *Health Affairs, 29*(2), 312–317. https://doi.org/10.1377/hlthaff.2009.0966

Mor, V., Leone, T., Maresso, A., (Eds.). (2014). *Regulating long-term care quality: An international comparison.* Cambridge University Press. isbn: 9781107665354.

Mor, V., Zinn, J., Angelelli, J., Teno, J. M., & Miller, S. C. (2004). Driven to tiers: Socioeconomic and racial disparities in the quality of nursing home care. *The Milbank Quarterly, 82*(2), 227–256. https://doi.org/10.1111/j.0887-378X.2004.00309.x

National Consumer Voice for Quality Long-Term Care. (2011, October). *10 no-cost ideas to advance your culture change journey by involving residents and families.* Retrieved from: https://www.google.com/url?client=internal-element-cse&cx=011469937775421039183:xqqhuix93jk&q=http://theconsumervoice.org/uploads/files/advocate/10-No-Cost-CC-Ideas-FINAL.pdf&sa=U&ved=2ahUKEwi6orPb_qn0AhXDpnIEHQDACMEQFnoECAAQAQ&usg=AOvVaw3cJNOoo38tMpugO-Au8FQ4.

Naumann, E. (1995). *Customer satisfaction measurement and management: Using the voice of the customer.* Thomson Executive Press.

Palmer, J., Eidson, V., Haliemun, C., & Wiewel, P. (2011). Predictors of positive and negative word of mouth of university students: Strategic implications for institutions of higher education. *International Journal of Business and Social Science, 2*(7), 59–62.

Pearson, A., Hocking, S., Mott, S., & Riggs, A. (1993). Quality of care in nursing homes: From the resident's perspective. *Journal of Advanced Nursing, 18*(1), 20–24. https://doi.org/10.1046/j.1365-2648.1993.18010020.x

Rantz, M. J., Hicks, L., Grando, V., Petroski, G. F., Madsen, R. W., Mehr, D. R., Conn, V., Zwygart-Staffacher, M., Scott, J., Flesner, M., Bostick, J., Porter, R., & Maas, M. (2004). Nursing home quality, cost, staffing, and staff mix. *The Gerontologist, 44*(1), 24–38. https://doi.org/10.1093/geront/44.1.24

Ratcliffe, J., Lester, L. H., Couzner, L., & Crotty, M. (2013). An assessment of the relationship between informal caring and quality of life in older community-dwelling adults – More positives than negatives? *Health and Social Care in the Community, 21*(1), 35–46. https://doi.org/10.1111/j.1365-2524.2012.01085.x

Sarvimaki, A., & Stenbock-Hult, B. (2000). Quality of life in old age described as a sense of Well-being, meaning and value. *Journal of Advanced Nursing, 32*(4), 1025–1033.

Schenk, L., Meyer, R., Behr, A., Kuhlmey, A., & Holzhausen, M. (2013). Quality of life in nursing homes: Results of a qualitative resident survey. *Quality of Life Research, 22*(10), 2929–2938. https://doi.org/10.1007/s11136-013-0400-2

Shin, J. H., & Hyun, T. K. (2015). Nurse staffing and quality of care of nursing home residents in Korea. *Journal of Nursing Scholarship, 47*(6), 555–564. https://doi.org/10.1111/jnu.12166

Shippee, T. P., Henning-Smith, C., Kane, R. L., & Lewis, T. (2015). Resident- and facility-level predictors of quality of life in long-term care. *The Gerontologist, 55*(4), 643–655. https://doi.org/10.1093/geront/gnt148

Stevenson, D. G. (2006). Nursing home consumer complaints and quality of care: A national view. *Medical Care Research and Review, 63*(3), 347–368. https://doi.org/10.1177/1077558706287043

Svensson, T. (1991). Intellectual exercise and quality of life in the frail elderly. In J. E. Birren, D. Deutchman, J. E. Lubben, & J. Rowe (Eds.), *The concept and measurement of quality of life in the frail elderly*. Academic Press.

Tilden, V. P., Tolle, S., Drach, L., & Hickman, S. (2002). Measurement of quality of care and quality of life at the end of life. *The Gerontologist, 42*(Suppl. 3), 71–80. https://doi.org/10.1093/geront/42.suppl_3.71

United Nations, Department of Economic and Social Affairs. (2019). *World population ageing 2019*. Retrieved from https://www.un.org/en/development/desa/population/publications/pdf/ageing/WorldPopulationAgeing2019-Highlights.pdf

United Nations, Department of Economic and Social Affairs. (2020). *Population dynamics: world population prospects 2019*. Retrieved from https://population.un.org/wpp/Graphs/Probabilistic/POP/65plus/900.

United States Census Bureau. (2014). *Fueled by aging baby boomers, nation's older population to nearly double in the next 20 years, census bureau reports*. Retrieved from https://www.census.gov/newsroom/press-releases/2014/cb14-84.html#:~:text=The%20nation's%2065%2Dand%2Dolder,from%20the%20U.S.%20Census%20Bureau.

United States Census Bureau. (2020). *2019 population estimates by age, sex, race and hispanic origin*. Retrieved from https://www.census.gov/newsroom/press-kits/2020/population-estimates-detailed.html.

Vaarama, M. (2009). Care-related quality of life in old age. *European Journal of Ageing, 6*, 113–125. https://doi.org/10.1007/s10433-009-0115-y

Vanleerberghe, P., De Witte, N., Claes, C., Schalock, R. L., & Verte, D. (2017). The quality of life of older people aging in place: A literature review. *Quality of Life Research, 26*(11), 2899–2907. https://doi.org/10.1007/s11136-017-1651-0

WeDO: European Partnership for the Wellbeing and Dignity of Older People. (2012). *European quality framework for long-term care services*. Retrieved from https://www.age-platform.eu/sites/default/files/EU_Quality_Framework_for_LTC-EN.pdf.

World Health Organization. (1946). Constitution. *American Journal of Public Health and the Nations Health, 36*, 1315–1323. https://doi.org/10.2105/AJPH.36.11.1315

Zimmerman, D. R. (2003). Improving nursing home quality of care through outcomes data: The MDS quality indicators. *International Journal of Geriatric Psychiatry, 18*(3), 250–257. https://doi.org/10.1002/gps.820

Chapter 2
Resident Autonomy, Dignity, and Respect

*I've learned that people will forget what you said, people will
forget what you did, but people will never forget how you
made them feel.* – Maya Angelou

Abstract All care recipients have an essential right to be treated as individuals.
From a moral imperative to the regulations governing the operations of long-term
care facilities, there are specific provisions related to resident dignity, autonomy and
choice, respect, privacy (when and to the extent possible), and individualization of
the care and services provided, each of which will be covered in turn. As part of
resident autonomy, this chapter covers resident councils, as well as the many ways in
which facility staff and leadership can and must engage with residents to support
them in directing their own care, thereby maximizing resident quality of life.
Additionally, research exploring residents' sense of purpose and how long-term
care facilities can enhance residents' feelings of self-worth and usefulness in congregate living settings is examined. Methods to promote a sense of purpose will be
addressed, which helps residents experience meaning and improves overall satisfaction and quality of life in long-term care.

Keywords Respect · Relationships · Care planning · Quality of life · Satisfaction ·
Autonomy · Self-determination · Dignity · Personal identity · Sense of purpose ·
Meaning · Service · Activities · Golden rule · Individuality · Control · Technology ·
Active participation

The premise of person-centered care is rooted in encompassing the fundamental
needs of care recipients—beyond their physical needs, also meeting their psychosocial and relational needs (Bagnasco et al., 2020). All people need to have autonomy and experience dignity to feel human, so long-term care residents should be
treated with dignity and respect and encouraged to exert their autonomy whenever
possible. Autonomy is a self-directed *action* that refers to self-determination and an
ability to exert control over one's life. In the context of long-term care, autonomy can
be challenging due to care recipients being dependent on others for assistance,

J. L. Johs-Artisensi, K. E. Hansen, *Quality of Life and Well-Being for Residents
in Long-Term Care Communities*, Human Well-Being Research and Policy Making,
https://doi.org/10.1007/978-3-031-04695-7_2

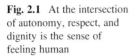
Fig. 2.1 At the intersection
of autonomy, respect, and
dignity is the sense of
feeling human

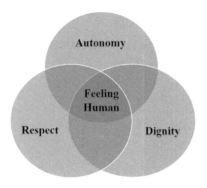

unable to do certain things for themselves, although many opportunities to support
and encourage individuals' autonomy still exist. Dignity is a *feeling* of being valued,
and psychologically comfortable. Respect is reciprocal and is effected as an *action*,
influencing the way one treats themselves and others. Additionally, the level at
which others' behavior toward someone is perceived as respectful (or not) will
evoke *feelings* in them, as well. There is a great deal of overlap and intersectionality
between these concepts, with the use of or level of one often influencing another,
ultimately impacting individuals' human experience (Fig. 2.1).

2.1   Respect

Respect can be difficult to define. It is demonstrated in the context of relationships
but may most easily be recognized in its absence. In various circumstances there are
different requirements for respect, but basic social guidelines include simple things
such as displaying courtesy and kindness, listening to others, acknowledging them,
honoring their sensitivities, and encouraging them to express ideas—essentially,
seeing them and treating them like people. One such way to respect residents is to
incorporate their preferences into care plans, as shown in Exhibit 2.1. In health care,
respect is an essential right of care recipients (World Health Organization, 2015),
and treating patients with respect is a cornerstone of nursing care (Koskenniemi
et al., 2019). Long-term care recipients should be treated in accordance with these
basic social guidelines to maintain their dignity, but another important way of
showing respect is by supporting residents in exerting their autonomy. At the core
of person-centered care is the integration of care recipients' viewpoints and involvement in their own care planning (World Health Organization, 2015), and doing so
demonstrates respect.

Exhibit 2.1 Preferences for Everyday Living Inventory (PELI)

The PELI is a freely available tool providers can use to help integrate care recipients' preferences into care planning. There are several versions of the tool (e.g. longer, shorter, LGBT-focused) to best suit provider and resident needs. Understanding and meeting care recipients' preferences, using a tool like PELI, will:

- Enhance nursing home residents' autonomy, quality of life, and physical and emotional well-being.
- Support more holistic care planning.
- Increase satisfaction among residents and their family members.
- Strengthen trust and communication among residents, family members and nursing home staff.
- Facilitate compliance with regulations requiring that care plans reflect residents' voices and preferences so each person can experience a meaningful and enjoyable life.

Adapted from Preference Based Living's "Integrating Preferences into Care Plans" (Humes et al., 2020).

Care recipients feeling respected by nursing staff is essential to their quality of life (Koskenniemi et al., 2015). There is a strong correlation between perceived respect and satisfaction with care (Koskenniemi et al., 2019), and most patient complaints are about disrespectful communication and behavior from staff (Reader, 2014). By treating residents with respect, departures from appropriate standards of care can be avoided and care deficiencies can be significantly reduced (Oosterveld-Vlug et al., 2014). Samples of caregiver behavior demonstrating respect can be found in Exhibit 2.2. Care recipients with the greatest care needs and highest levels of dependency often report the lowest levels of perceived respect (Koskenniemi et al., 2019). This underscores the importance of staff exhibiting caring attitudes, sensitivity, and attentiveness, especially to those who rely on them the most.

Exhibit 2.2 10 Ways Caregivers Can Show Care Recipients Respect

1. Treat every care recipient equally.
2. Remember basic courtesies.
3. Be present with your care recipient.
4. Get acquainted.
5. Understand the care recipient's perspective.
6. Communicate with respect.
7. Replace labeling with positive solutions.
8. Keep personal conversations out of earshot.

(continued)

Exhibit 2.2 (continued)
  9. Support a healthy work environment.
  10. Attend to your own well-being.

  *Adapted from American Mobile's "10 Ways to ensure respectful care of ICU patients" (*Wood, 2016*).*

2.2 Autonomy

When seniors move into long-term care communities, they leave the familiarity of their surroundings and routines behind and may experience a loss of control (McCabe et al., 2021). To ensure safe and efficient care, some care centers structure policies, schedules, and routines (Lan, 2017) that can make it difficult for residents' autonomy to be preserved (Carter & Van Puymbroeck, 2010). Autonomy refers to people's ability to make meaningful decisions for themselves and, in doing so, direct the course of their life, care, and well-being. It allows each individual to recognize their personal needs and goals and have a sense of control over their own life (Hertz, 1996) (Fig. 2.2).

Residents' quality of life is influenced by their perception of autonomy (Johs-Artisensi et al., 2020), because personal control plays a major role in social and emotional well-being (Carter & Van Puymbroeck, 2010). Resident choice in care tasks such as dressing, where in the building they spend their time, morning and bedtime routines, and socializing are all significant predictors of quality of life (McCabe et al., 2021). Residents afforded more choice report higher life satisfaction (Bangerter, 2017), feel enhanced respect and dignity, and experience increased feelings of usefulness, value, and life satisfaction (Liu et al., 2020). When residents have a sense of control, they feel more independent, develop confidence, and improve their well-being (Carter & Van Puymbroeck, 2010).

Fostering autonomy is essential in long-term care because it fuels self-determination and intrinsic motivation, leading residents to be more engaged, participate in activities, ward off depressive symptoms, and improve their quality of life (Carter & Van Puymbroeck, 2010). Making choices boosts residents' value, self-respect, and dignity (Liu et al., 2020). However, when autonomy is lacking, residents risk losing self-esteem, developing learned helplessness, and further losing their independence (Carter & Van Puymbroeck, 2010), potentially decreasing participation in therapy or treatment programs, activities, and events, and leaving them more isolated. The more residents experience these negative consequences and feelings, the more withdrawn they may become, perpetuating a negative spiral that decreases quality of life.

Most long-term care recipients are dependent, to some degree, on assistance for their activities of daily living or mobility needs (Liu et al., 2020) (Fig. 2.3). Although this diminished functional capacity can be a barrier (Tuominen et al., 2016), care recipients still desire autonomy (Welford, 2012). In fact, autonomy mediates the

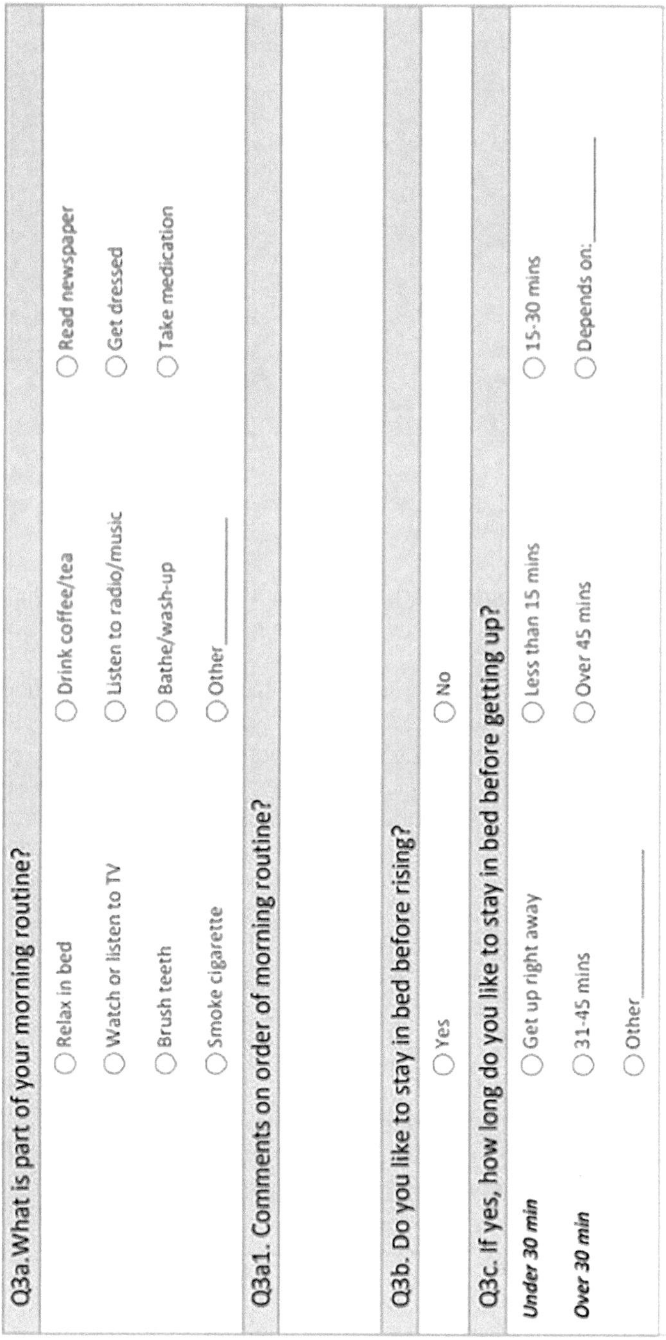

Q3a. What is part of your morning routine?

- ◯ Relax in bed
- ◯ Drink coffee/tea
- ◯ Read newspaper
- ◯ Watch or listen to TV
- ◯ Listen to radio/music
- ◯ Get dressed
- ◯ Brush teeth
- ◯ Bathe/wash-up
- ◯ Take medication
- ◯ Smoke cigarette
- ◯ Other _____

Q3a1. Comments on order of morning routine?

Q3b. Do you like to stay in bed before rising?

- ◯ Yes
- ◯ No

Q3c. If yes, how long do you like to stay in bed before getting up?

Under 30 min
- ◯ Get up right away
- ◯ Less than 15 mins
- ◯ 15-30 mins

Over 30 min
- ◯ 31-45 mins
- ◯ Over 45 mins
- ◯ Depends on: _____
- ◯ Other _____

Fig. 2.2 Excerpt from the Preferences for Everyday Living Inventory (PELI)—Nursing Home version. Developed by Kimberly van Haitsma (2019) (CC BY-ND 4.0)

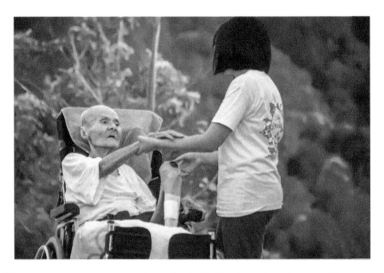

Fig. 2.3 A caregiver assists a resident who is highly dependent for care. The more highly dependent for care long-term care residents are, the more reliant they are on caregivers to facilitate their autonomy. Photo Credit: Truth Seeker

relationship between functional ability and life satisfaction, so even in the face of physical impairments, when efforts are made to increase autonomy, life satisfaction increases (Liu et al., 2020).

Person-centered care prioritizes residents' dignity by allowing them self-determination when incorporating their needs and preferences into their care plans. This is based on self-determination theory, as shown in Exhibit 2.3. A key pathway to ensuring residents have a say in their daily routines and care activities is supporting strong resident-staff relationships (Degenholtz, 2014). Resident-staff relationships and autonomy are two of the largest contributors to and predictors of quality of life (Johs-Artisensi et al., 2020; McCabe et al., 2021). Ironically, when residents are more dependent on staff for their care, the involvement of others is required to promote their autonomy and free will, which is what residents want and need. Many residents are unhappy with their level of autonomy and decisional control (Boyle, 2004), specifically desiring to have greater control over their care routines and an ability to leave the care community (Kane et al., 1997).

Exhibit 2.3 Self-Determination Theory
Self-Determination theory suggests people are able to become self-determined (motivated to grow and change) when three key needs are fulfilled:

- Competence.
- Connection.
- Autonomy.

(continued)

Exhibit 2.3 (continued)
*Adapted from Verywell Mind's "Self-Determination Theory and Motivation" (*Cherry, 2021*).*

2.3 Dignity

In a civilized society, it is often considered a moral imperative and a human right to be treated with dignity and respect, and the concept of how dignity applies to the treatment of older adults in long-term care communities has been extensively studied (e.g., Kane & de Vries, 2017). Although the concept of dignity is multifaceted, the aspect which applies most closely to long-term care recipients, who are dependent on others, is the notion of *dignity of personal identity* (Nordenfelt & Edgar, 2005). This relates to a person's self-esteem; is comprised of integrity, autonomy, and inclusion; and can be endangered and disrupted if residents are not treated as unique human beings. As dependency increases, autonomy is at risk, and the loss of choice and control is closely linked to dignity (Kane & de Vries, 2017). Beyond the loss of autonomy, other ways in which dignity can be violated include: (a) not being seen, (b) being seen only as a member of a group rather than as a unique individual, (c) breaches of personal space, and (d) humiliation (Mann, 1998). Some rights of residents designed to preserve dignity are shown in Exhibit 2.4. Care recipients in long-term care communities are at risk of experiencing loss of dignity in all of these areas (Kisvetrova, 2019).

Exhibit 2.4 Nursing Home Residents' Rights
In the United States in 1987, as part of the Nursing Home Reform Act (OBRA 1987), nursing home residents were granted a list of rights, which stress the importance of individual dignity and self-determination.
  These include the right to:

- Be treated with respect.
- Participate in activities.
- Be free from discrimination.
- Be free from abuse and neglect.
- Be free from restraints.
- Make complaints.
- Get proper medical care.
- Have their representative notified.
- Get information on services and fees.
- Manage one's own money.
- Get proper privacy, property, and living arrangements.

(continued)

Exhibit 2.4 (continued)
- Spend time with visitors.
- Get social services.
- Leave the nursing home.
- Have protection against unfair transfer or discharge.
- Form or participate in resident groups.
- Have family and friends involved in care and services.

Adapted from the Center for Medicare and Medicaid Services' "Your Rights and Protections as a Nursing Home Resident".

The provision of dignified care and services is crucial for maintaining care recipients' quality of life (World Health Organization, 2011). When a resident's dignity is preserved, it strengthens their life spirit—an inner sense of freedom, self-respect, and successful coping (Anderberg, 2007). Having dignity reduces residents' feelings of uselessness and lacking value (Liu et al., 2020) and enhances life satisfaction (Burack, 2012). In contrast, when care recipients are treated in ways that cause them to lose their dignity, deleterious effects follow, including loss of self-determination and control; feelings of their personal lives or space being violated; and negative emotional states of sadness, hopelessness, and worthlessness. Residents may become socially disconnected and experience increased concern about being a burden on others (Staats et al., 2020). When dignity is fractured, it can be associated with depression and even a desire for death (Chochinov et al., 2002).

Residents of long-term care communities are at particular risk of losing dignity because of their vulnerability, not only because they're functionally incapacitated, which can threaten their perceptions of self and leaves them dependent on others for care, but because they also lack social support (Oosterveld-Vlug et al., 2014). Thus, it is imperative that long-term care providers are educated and well-trained in the provision of dignity-preserving care.

2.4   Sense of Purpose

Having a sense of purpose in life is fundamental to human beings (Dragaset et al., 2017). People find purpose in many ways, including through creative works, performing meaningful tasks, and having someone to love and care about (Frankl, 1963). Examples of how some nursing home residents defined sense of purpose are found in Exhibit 2.5. Although a concept less studied among long-term care recipients, there seems to be a participatory and intentional nature associated with many key contributors to nursing home residents' quality of life. For example, residents cite the importance of relationships and a sense of community—which are of an active, reciprocal nature—and contributory service, where they embrace engaging roles and responsibilities which give them a sense of purpose (Johs-Artisensi et al.,

2020). Through relationships and contributions, residents value the opportunity to make a positive difference in others' lives.

Exhibit 2.5 How Nursing Home Residents Find Sense of Purpose: In Their Own Words

As part of a research study, nursing home residents were asked what contributed to their sense of purpose. The top five categories that best encapsulated their responses included (in order of importance): Sense of community, Activities, Communication with family members, Contributory service to the care community, and Quality of care. Some of the residents' individual responses included:

I get everyone involved and they fill me in on whatever is going on. They don't call me the mayor for nothing.

I attend activities, write poems for people in the facility, and enjoy being a part of resident council—we help get changes made around here.

I use my energy to be an upbeat light to everyone here. I really think I make a difference in some of these people's lives. Now they talk to me, and say hello to me when I'm walking down the hall.

I like to make birthday cards for everyone.

Adapted from "Qualitative and Quantitative Analysis of Quality of Life Survey Results Research Report" (Hansen et al., 2018).

A sense of purpose is an important predictor of quality of life (O'Rourke, 2015). When care recipients have opportunities to engage in purposeful occupational tasks in the long-term care community, such activity fosters feelings of dignity and gives them a sense of satisfaction (O'Sullivan & Hocking, 2006). Participation in meaningful activities promotes physical activity, social stimulation, and personal identity, all of which can slow age-related decline. However, when deprived of meaningful and purposeful opportunities, both residents' health and well-being are negatively impacted (Slettebø et al., 2017).

2.5 Promoting Respect, Autonomy, Purpose, and Dignity in Residential Care Communities

Having considered dignity, respect, autonomy, and purpose, as well as their inter-related nature, it is clear that by treating residents with respect, supporting their autonomy, and fueling their purpose, caregivers can best support residents in experiencing dignity in long-term care communities. Staff are the cornerstone of care, and to meet the fundamental physical, relational, and psychosocial care needs of residents, they must be supported in providing quality care. This means they need education and training around the philosophy of care, expectations about their behavior and actions, and adequate time to provide resident care, as without it, staff may prioritize physical needs and, as a result, care recipients' quality of life can suffer. To ensure long-term care recipients have dignity and purpose, they must be treated with respect and their autonomy must be supported. In fact, this is an element of care that consumers will increasingly demand. Many care recipients indeed have a choice about where and how to receive care, and if one care center is not affording residents dignity, respect, and autonomy, their competitor certainly will.

2.5.1 The Golden Rule

Appropriate care and services for residents could probably be summed up in a single sentence—"Treat others the way you'd like to be treated"—or, in an even shorter phrase—"Be nice." It is a simple premise but, pragmatically, often more difficult to accomplish than it should be. All who work in the care community should ensure their interactions with care recipients are polite and respectful. Many strategies discussed here also can aid staff members in treating residents respectfully but, beyond simple good manners, showing respect includes respecting residents' privacy and personal space. Staff should also be sensitive to and inclusive with residents and treat them as customers, not as burdens. A term encompassing many of these principles that has recently come into use in health and long-term care settings is "hospitality" (Johs-Artisensi et al., 2021). Hospitality practices in residential care settings include care recipients being given a warm welcome upon admission, staff anticipating and meeting their needs and wants through individually tailored care plans, and providing residents a comfortable environment (Fig. 2.4).

Residents should be shown they are valued as individuals, by hearing them, seeing them, and relating to them. Residents need to receive attention from people. Staff, friends, and family should connect with care recipients, ask them questions, show an interest in their lives from the past and the present, and solicit their opinions whenever and wherever possible. Staff focusing on optimizing resident quality of life can look for ways to share joyful moments with residents, such as congratulating

Fig. 2.4 While the "golden rule" often applies to staff members, residents can be a beacon of positive support and advocacy for each other, as well. Photo Credit: Eberhard Grossgasteiger

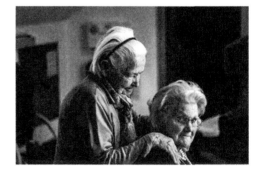

when a new great-grandson is born or when a granddaughter gets married. By acknowledging the event, staff boost the resident's joy, which increases their well-being. Residents need to be actively listened to and validated as human beings through daily interactions with various staff members at the care center. This can be done by verbally reflecting the resident's thoughts back, to show them they have been heard. If a resident has made a request or complaint, it shows respect to follow up with them in a timely manner to resolve the matter. Residents also need to be provided with information so they can understand what's happening around them. They deserve to have explanations about what, when, and why a decision has been made or something is happening, even in the presence of cognitive impairments. Especially for care recipients who are physically dependent for care, if a procedure is being done to them, such as transferring their body in a mechanical lift, a step-by-step narration of what exactly is happening to them will help them to feel more at ease and less out of control.

Finally, residents want and deserve to be acknowledged. Respect and dignity flow from acknowledgement, as noted in Exhibit 2.6. Staff should address care recipients by their preferred name and help them to see ways in which they remain capable and confident in their everyday lives. Staff can compliment residents on their appearance, on a craft project or puzzle that's been completed, or on a sweet gesture they saw the resident make for a friend. Residents also appreciate being recognized for contributions they make to the care community or for extra efforts they put in to making it a better place to live. The active exchange of these acknowledgments reinforces residents' self-value and sense of belonging within the community.

Exhibit 2.6 Acknowledging Care Recipients Shows Dignity and Respect

All care recipients deserve to be treated with dignity, respect, and an acknowledgment of their value as individuals. One of the most widely cited elements of disrespect mentioned by residents is simply failing to pay attention to their needs, by leaving them unattended or ignored. This translates to the resident experience in the way they are greeted at admission, as nurse aides are performing daily cares, or if they are wandering in the hall. The building is "home" to the residents, and in many ways, employees are guests in their lives and should act accordingly.

This is demonstrated by listening to residents, asking for their opinions, and recognizing the importance of incorporating their personal values and preferences into the way care is provided. Respect is conveyed by being considerate of residents' time (e.g., striving to provide timely service and apologizing when we fail to do so). The physical environment created for care recipients is a direct reflection of our respect for them—the ability to ensure privacy, cleanliness and quiet surroundings speaks volumes. When staff request permission to enter a resident's room, ask them how they would like to be addressed, and caregivers explain to residents who they are and what they

(continued)

Exhibit 2.6 (continued)
plan to do, this all communicates respect for residents as individuals. Respect is also showing gratitude to residents who entrust us with their care. A simple thank you can mean so much.
   Adapted from Harvard Medical School's "Setting the Stage: Why Health Care Needs a Culture of Respect" (James, 2018)

2.5.2   Autonomy, Choice, and Control

When care recipients make their own choice about moving into a long-term care community, they tend to be happier than those who felt forced into the decision (Reinardy, 1995), but even when only given choice or control over an *element* of something, positive benefits ensue. Most care recipients would not elect to have the illnesses or disabilities they have and would prefer to live independently, so especially given the lack of choice in those matters, finding ways their autonomy *can* be supported is paramount. In many cases, residents can be offered options regarding their schedules—what they want to do and when. Even if those options are limited, perhaps they can be given choices about how or where something will occur, or who they will be with. Consider assistance with activities of daily living—in terms of dressing, care recipients should have control over when they want to get up and get dressed for the day and what they want to wear. When it comes to bathing, residents can be offered choices about which day or time of day they would like to be bathed, whether they prefer a bath or a shower, whether they want to wash their hair first or last, what scent of shampoo or soap they like to use, or whether they would like their towel to be warmed. Residents should also be given options relative to the dining experience, as shown in Exhibit 2.7. This is expanded on more in the Food and Dining chapter, but to encourage autonomy, residents should have some choice in what they eat and when. Some facilities have moved away from fixed mealtimes to more flexible dining schedules, giving residents more alternatives for when they want to eat, or various options to obtain a meal or a snack outside of scheduled meal periods. Residents should also be given at least some options of food choices, and they need to be made aware of such choices—if a kitchen is willing to provide an alternative entrée if the resident asks for it, that should be communicated as an option versus only something that is honored as a special request, and ideally choices should be able to be made as close to the point of service as possible. Residents should also be offered options regarding where they want to eat (e.g., in their own room or in the dining room with peers) and who they want to eat with, as mealtimes can be an excellent opportunity to facilitate social relationships.

Exhibit 2.7 Baby Boomers: The "Food Court" Generation

Abbey Delray South, a Florida retirement community, involved its residents in a redesign of their food service. What was once a cafeteria-style dining room with a salad bar was transformed into a formal dining room, a bistro with a grab-and-go section, and an entry lounge that serves food. The ability to eat outdoors or reserve a private room for meals or parties was also included, and the enhanced dining program was supported with new training for kitchen staff and servers.

Leadership recognized that Baby Boomers had high expectations for food—they jokingly referred to them as the "food court" generation—as they are accustomed to having multiple choices, including when and what to eat, which is exactly what this retirement community wanted to accommodate by offering alternate dining approaches. Even the once narrow corridor leading to the dining room was remodeled, creating a more gracious entry. The dining experience was clearly one of the main social engagements residents had each day, so accoutrements such as colored tablecloths and napkins, programs like theme nights, and special events like wine tastings, were added to help keep their new dining experience vibrant.

Adapted from McKnight's Long-Term Living News' "Dining Upgrades a la 'Cart'" (Surico, 2014).

Care recipients' active involvement in the care planning process is vital to supporting their autonomy and their participation serves to improve their satisfaction with care and services. When staff know residents and what is important to them well, staff can integrate residents' needs, wishes, interests, and preferences into an individualized care plan unique to each person. Ideally, a balance can be struck whereby a care plan captures the general preferences of the resident, while still encouraging them to exercise their autonomy throughout all their daily interactions, as described above.

Care recipients should be involved in their therapeutic treatments, too. Residents should always be included in decision-making about therapies or treatment options and given adequate information to ensure they are providing informed consent, as well as be given the option to decline treatment. Preferably, care recipients should also have some say in when therapies or treatments are scheduled. For example, if they find cognitive therapies more exhausting than physical therapies, they may have a preference about the order of their therapies. Additionally, therapies should be scheduled around other activities that are important to the resident, so they don't have to miss out on enriching psychosocial opportunities.

Residents also need to be given opportunities for education and to learn new things. Many care recipients may be new to fast-changing technology, but if given the proper education and support, they may find that using technology such as a tablet device or an automated assistant (e.g., Amazon Alexa or Apple's Siri, noted in Exhibit 2.8) gives them much more autonomy to stay close to friends and family outside the care community, stay connected to the world and learn new things, or even to achieve newfound independence with the ability to "ask Alexa" what the weather is, whether their favorite sports team won their game, or to play a nostalgic song. Whether it is technology-assisted or not, increased independence, autonomy, and control will boost residents' self-determination and satisfaction. Another way to facilitate independence, purpose, and autonomy is to promote restorative care and physical fitness opportunities, because with less functional impairment, it is easier for residents to exert autonomy more independently.

> **Exhibit 2.8 Voice Assistants Offer Seniors Autonomy, Independence, and Social Connection**
> As voice recognition technologies become more inexpensive and accessible, long-term care communities have taken notice of the promises such devices may hold for offering older adults greater independence and social connection.
> The Front Porch Center for Innovation and Wellbeing worked with Carlsbad By The Sea, a California retirement community, to launch a six-month Amazon Alexa pilot study with a group of residents, largely in their 80s. Residents attended twice-monthly "Alexa 101" workshops, and technicians helped users customize their devices based on individual interests. Overall, participants felt that Alexa made their lives easier, with 75% using it at least once a day – mostly to check the weather, hear the latest news, listen to music, search for information, or set a timer. The majority also reported feeling more connected to family, friends, and the community, including some who used Alexa to call their loved ones. Researchers were excited about how voice assistants can be a powerful tool to help older adults live well and were impressed with the energy and enthusiasm older adults had for the technology.
> *Adapted from McKnight's Long-Term Care News' "Voice Assistants Finding Niche with Elders" (Novotney, 2018)*

Autonomy and choice must also be prevalent in the provision of meaningful opportunities for residents, and this is easily achievable. The chapter on Activities and Religious Practices contains more detail on providing meaningful activities, but thoughtful providers will be intentional in specifically promoting resident autonomy, dignity, and sense of purpose. Autonomy in activities is beneficial, because when residents are empowered to choose how to spend their time and are supported in their choices, they become active and engaged members of a care community. Active participation helps time pass more quickly plus, when residents choose activities that are meaningful, purposeful, or important to their identity, their competence and self-esteem grows, increasing motivation for future engagement and creating a positive cycle. A variety of activities should be offered so that residents can choose to participate in those they have enjoyed in the past as well as options to explore new things. Residents may appreciate the predictability of regularly scheduled activities, as well as the interspersing of novel events. Residents should be asked for suggestions about what activities they would like to have available and be included in the planning processes for upcoming events, so they have experiences to look forward to and engage with fellow members of the care center. It is also important for residents to be able to choose alone time or disengagement, too, as some may prefer solitude for rest, reflection, or contemplation. Additionally, a resident's desire to change their mind must also be respected—their health status may change, they may be more fatigued, or they may simply want to try something new. However, staff should also be wary of depressive symptoms, to ensure they can be addressed and treated in a timely manner. Sometimes supporting autonomy in the face of depression, which can alter mood, motivation, and experiences of joy, can be a difficult balance, as depressed care recipients may need additional coaxing toward engagement activities as part of their treatment.

To further promote autonomy and purpose for residents with higher levels of independence, opportunities to help plan and then attend field trips or community outings can be stimulating and engaging. By making suggestions for activities or events and helping to make the plans, residents are participating in creating experiences which they can look forward to, will bring them joy, and will lead to new memories. Even within the care community, for residents who are able, offering them responsibilities such as watering plants, delivering mail, setting up crafts, or connecting people—assisting those with disabilities, cheering up a friend, or welcoming a new resident—are all activities that can offer residents a significant sense of purpose and a role in cultivating the community itself.

Residents likely also have ideas and opinions about the culture and operations of their care communities and may appreciate the opportunity to share their level of satisfaction or voice concerns or compliments about community happenings. One meaningful way to ensure the collective voice of residents is heard is through the provision of a resident council, a structured group meeting that allows residents to voice their needs and present suggestions. Rationale for strengthening existing resident councils is shown in Exhibit 2.9. Such councils are especially effective when a dedicated staff member is assigned as a liaison to the group to respond to their concerns and inquiries. Resident councils not only offer care recipients an avenue through which they can advocate and effect change for themselves and their peers, but may lead to changes that positively affect residents' lives while strengthening participants' sense of purpose as active and engaged members of their care communities.

Exhibit 2.9 Three Reasons to Strengthen your Resident Council
Residents tell it like it is—Residents are more likely to speak up than the average staff member because they're not worried about losing their jobs. Residents will tell you what you need to know to make your facility shine enough to attract more residents.

(continued)

Exhibit 2.9 (continued)

Free labor—While employees are running around short-staffed, residents often find the opportunity to do something interesting very appealing. Care communities are full of diverse, experienced, motivated, and sometimes bored individuals yearning to have a sense of purpose. They may need assistance, but working together they can effect positive change. Maybe they could raise money to contribute toward an herb garden for the patio or start a welcoming committee to reduce isolation of new residents. Their ideas may be exactly what's needed to revitalize demoralized staff members and energize your institution.

A marketing goldmine—That herb garden is going to brighten the faces of new prospects touring your establishment. And when you tell them it was conceived of and designed by residents? That's exactly what people want—to be an active part of the community despite their health challenges.

Adapted from McKnight's Long-Term Living News' "3 Surprising Reasons to Strengthen Your Resident Council" (Barbera, 2016).

For residents experiencing cognitive impairment, offering choices remains important but should be done in a manner the person can comprehend without stress or fear of incapability. Family members can be useful proxies in discerning the interests and likely preferences of those who may be unable to remember or communicate for themselves. One suggestion, which is good for all residents but may be especially suitable for cognitively impaired residents, includes celebrating holidays or other cultural events. Traditional events that have been celebrated many times in the past are likely to evoke fond memories and feelings, especially if family are included in these events. Another meaningful activity is personal storytelling. The process of sitting down with someone to listen to and engage with their stories allows the care recipient to be an active participant in their own life and relay important events to others. Residents will feel heard and valued, and it allows caregivers to learn more about their life and who they are as a person.

Finally, ensuring residents have ample opportunity to maintain and develop trusting relationships with family, friends, peers, and staff is critical to supporting their care and preserving their dignity and sense of purpose. Detailed practices to cultivate these varied relationships are discussed further in the Relationships with Other Residents, Staff, and Family Members chapter but, in short, staff need adequate time to learn and honor the essence of each resident in their care. Staff or volunteers can engage residents in activities, whether simple conversations or asking questions, sharing a cup of coffee or a meal, or joining on an outing. Care communities can support residents' connections with friends and families by inviting them to participate in care community events. Additionally, staff can play a "matchmaker" role in introducing and connecting residents with common interests to promote friendships. Staff can also empower residents and acknowledge them for the ways

Fig. 2.5 Connecting with care recipients honors their essence, helping them feel value and self-worth. Photo Credit: Truth Seeker

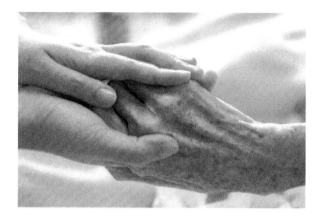

in which they help to bring the community to life through their social connections and unique contributions (Fig. 2.5).

2.6 Essential Influencers

Although every person within the care community should treat residents with whom they interact with dignity and respect, there are some key staff who play especially important roles in supporting resident-driven care and facilitating resident autonomy.

2.6.1 Nurses and Nurse Aides

Nurses and nurse aides are likely to have the most daily interaction with residents, although in care settings where care recipients have less acute medical needs, these personnel may not hold credentials with the word "nurse" in the title, and may instead be referred to as resident assistants, personal care workers, care attendants, or a variety of other titles. Regardless of nomenclature, the people who care recipients most rely on for care, support, and services, should always behave respectfully and hospitably in their interactions. They should be intentional in their relationship development with residents, getting to know who each resident is as a unique individual and cultivating an understanding of their interests and preferences. They should ensure residents' preferences are incorporated into care plans and regularly confirm that any individualized routines they have developed for residents remain in alignment with their current predilections. Nursing staff should also actively assist residents in exerting their autonomy throughout the day, throughout provision of services and supports, by engaging the resident and offering choices whenever possible.

2.6.2   Social Workers and Admissions Directors

Several types of individuals may hold positions related to social services within care centers. These are often social workers but may also include positions such as Admissions Director, Case Manager, or Care Coordinator. Like nursing staff, social workers should also be respectful and hospitable as they get to know residents, especially during the admissions process when a resident first arrives. Documenting a thorough inventory at the time of admission of the resident's past and current hobbies, interests, and preferences is critical to being able to craft an effective care plan and to individualize care and services in a way that promotes autonomy and dignity during their time at the care community. Social workers should also be attentive to regular monitoring of residents' moods and actively working to adjust treatment plans to ensure practices to support autonomy, purposeful activity, and relationship-building are included as part of any efforts to prevent or improve any negative mood symptoms. Social workers can be instrumental liaisons to both starting and supporting active resident councils.

2.6.3   Activities Directors and Aides

Staff within the activities department are tasked with meeting both the collective and individual needs of residents. By hospitably interacting with residents, they should be intentional about getting to know their personalities and interests. They should work to develop a wide variety of programming to meet the unique interests of the residents within their care community and be thoughtful about scheduling to ensure that residents are able to participate in activities of their choosing. Given that activities provide opportunities both for individual engagement and relationship development with peers, activities staff should take an intentional role in ensuring every resident can be engaged in meaningful and purposeful activities of their choosing. They should also actively involve residents and families to assist in planning novel events, both within the care community (e.g., holiday celebrations, cultural events) as well as opportunities for care recipients to join in activities outside and even within the local community at large, when possible.

2.6.4   Dietary Directors and Aides

The dining experience is highly important to residents, and a basic role to facilitate dignity and respect is to ensure food is of appropriate quality and served in a hospitable manner. Dining is also an area highly amenable to offering choice and autonomy, so directors should structure dining programs in such a way that residents are offered flexibility and choice in when, where, and what they eat for any given meal. Serving windows for scheduled meals should be expanded to allow for flexibility in timing, and a minimum of two choices should be offered and communicated for every meal, preferably at the point of service. Dietary aides or food servers should assist residents in understanding and making choices that suit their preferences.

References

Anderberg, P. L. M. (2007). Preserving dignity in caring for older adults: A concept analysis. *Journal of Advanced Nursing, 59*, 635–643.

Bagnasco, A., Zanini, M., Dasso, N., Rossi, S., Timmins, F., Galanti, C., … Sasso, L. (2020). Dignity, privacy, respect and choice—A scoping review of measurement of these concepts within acute healthcare practice. *Journal of Clinical Nursing, 29*, 1832–1857. https://doi.org/10.1111/jocn.15245

Bangerter, L. R. (2017). Honoring the everyday preferences of nursing home residents: Perceived choice and satisfaction with care. *The Gerontologist, 57*(3), 479–486. https://doi.org/10.1093/geront/gnv697

Barbera, E. F. (2016, October 11). *3 surprising reasons to strengthen your resident council.* McKnight's Long-Term Living News. https://www.mcknights.com/blogs/the-world-according-to-dr-el/3-surprising-reasons-to-strengthen-your-resident-council/

Boyle, G. (2004). Facilitating choice and control for older people in long-term care. *Health and Social Care in the Community, 12*(3), 212–220.

Burack, O. W. A. (2012). What matters most to nursing home elders: Quality of life in the nursing home. *Journal of the American Medical Directors Association, 13*(1), 48–53.

Carter, L., & Van Puymbroeck, M. (2010). The importance of autonomy in nursing home facilities. *American Journal of Recreation Therapy, 9*, 41–45. https://doi.org/10.5055/ajrt.2010.0013

Cherry, K. (2021, March 15). *Self-determination theory and motivation.* Verywell Mind. https://www.verywellmind.com/what-is-self-determination-theory-2795387.

Chochinov, H., Hack, T., Hassard, T., Kristjanson, L., McClement, S., & Harlos, M. (2002). Dignity in the terminally ill: A cross-sectional, cohort study. *Lancet, 360*(9350), 2026–2030.

Degenholtz, H. B. (2014). Mproving quality of life in nursing homes: The structured resident interview approach. *Journal of Aging Research, 2014*, 892679. https://doi.org/10.1155/2014/892679

Dragaset, J., Haugan, G., & Tranvag, O. (2017). Crucial aspects promoting meaning and purpose in life: Perceptions of nursing hone residents. *BMC Geriatrics, 17*(254), 1–9. https://doi.org/10.1186/s12877-017-0650-x

Frankl, V. (1963). *Man's search for meaning.* Washington Square Press.

Hansen, K. E., Johs-Artisensi, J. L., Olson, D., Berg, N., & Parker, K. (2018). *Qualitative and quantitative analysis of quality of life survey results research report.* Center for Health Administration and Aging Services Excellence.

Hertz, J. (1996). Conceptualization of perceived enactment of autonomy in the elderly. *Issues in Mental Health Nursing, 17*(3), 261–273. https://doi.org/10.3109/01612849609049919

Humes, S., Abbott, K., & Van Haitsma, K. (2020, October 2). *Integrating preferences into care plans.* Preference Based Living. https://www.preferencebasedliving.com/tip-sheets/integrating-preferences-into-care-plans/.

James, T. A. (2018, August 31). *Setting the stage: Why health care needs a culture of respect.* Harvard Medical School. https://postgraduateeducation.hms.harvard.edu/trends-medicine/setting-stage-why-health-care-needs-culture-respect.

Johs-Artisensi, J., Hansen, K., & Olson, D. (2020). Qualitative analyses of nursing home residents' quality of life from multiple stakeholders' perspectives. *Quality of Life Research, 29*(5), 1229–1238. https://doi.org/10.1007/s11136-019-02395-3

Johs-Artisensi, J., Hansen, K., Olson, D., & Creapeau, L. (2021). Leadership perceptions and practices of hospitality in senior care. *Journal of Applied Gerontology, 40*(6), 598–597. https://doi.org/10.1177/0733464820923903

Kane, R., Caplan, A., Urv-Wong, E., Freeman, C., Aroskar, M., & Finch, M. (1997). Everyday matters in the lives of nursing home residents: Wish for and perception of choice and control. *Journal of the American Geriatrics Society, 45*(9), 1086–1093.

Kane, J., & de Vries, K. (2017). Dignity in long-term care: An application of Nordenfelt's work. *Nursing Ethics, 24*(6), 744–751. https://doi.org/10.1177/0969733015624487

Kisvetrova, H. (2019). Dignity in old age. *Profese Online, 12*(2), 10–11. https://doi.org/10.5507/pol.2019.006

Koskenniemi, J., Leino-Kilpi, H., Puukka, P., & Suhonen, R. (2019). Respect and its associated factors as perceived by older patients. *Journal of Clinical Nursing, 28*, 3848–3857. https://doi.org/10.1111/jocn.15013

Koskenniemi, J., Leino-Kilpi, H., & Suhonen, R. (2015). Manifestation of respect in the care of older patients in long-term care settings. *Scandinavian Journal of Caring Sciences, 29*, 288–296. https://doi.org/10.1111/scs.12162

Lan, S. H. (2017). Educational intervention on physical restraint use in long-term care facilities— Systematic review and meta-analysis. *The Kaohsiung Journal of Medical Sciences, 33*(8), 411–421. https://doi.org/10.1016/j.kjms.2017.05.012

Liu, L., Kao, C., & Ying, J. (2020). Functional capacity and life satisfaction in older adult residents living in long-term care facilities: The mediator of autonomy. *The Journal of Nursing Research, 28*(4), 1–7.

Mann, J. (1998). The UDHR's revolutionary first article. *Health and Human Rights, 3*(2), 30–38.

McCabe, M., Byers, J., Lucy Busija, L., Mellor, D., Bennett, M., & Beattie, E. (2021). How important are choice, autonomy, and relationships in predicting the quality of life of nursing home residents? *Journal of Applied Gerontology, 40*(12), 1743–1750. https://doi.org/10.1177/0733464820983972

Nordenfelt, L., & Edgar, A. (2005). The four notions of dignity. *Quality in Ageing and Older Adults, 6*(1), 17–21. https://doi.org/10.1108/14717794200500004

Novotney, A. (2018, September 5). *Voice assistants finding niche with elders*. McKnight's Long-Term Care News. https://www.mcknights.com/news/voice-assistants-finding-niche-with-elders/.

O'Rourke, H. M. (2015). Factors that affect quality of life from the perspective of people with dementia: A metasynthesis. *Journal of the American Geriatrics Society, 63*(1), 24–38. https://doi.org/10.1111/jgs.13178

O'Sullivan, G., & Hocking, C. (2006). Positive ageing in residential care. *New Zealand Journal of Occupational Therapy, 53*, 17–23.

Oosterveld-Vlug, M., Pasman, H., van Gennip, I., Muller, M., Willems, D., & Onwuteaka-Philipsen, B. (2014). Dignity and the factors that influence it according to nursing home residents: A qualitative interview study. *Journal of Advanced Nursing, 70*, 97–106. https://doi.org/10.1111/jan.12171

Reader, T. W. (2014). Patient complaints in healthcare systems: A systematic review and coding taxonomy. *BMJ Quality and Safety, 23*, 678–689. https://doi.org/10.1136/bmjqs.2013-002437

Reinardy, J. (1995). Relocation to a new environment: Decisional control and the move to a nursing home. *Health and Social Work, 20*(1), 31–38.

Slettebø, Å., Sæteren, B., Caspari, S., Lohne, V., Rehnsfeldt, A., Heggestad, A., . . . Nåden, D. (2017). The significance of meaningful and enjoyable activities for nursing home resident's experiences of dignity. *Scandinavian Journal of Caring Sciences, 31*, 718–726. https://doi.org/10.1111/scs.12386

Staats, K., Grov, E., Husebo, B., & Tranvag, O. (2020). Dignity and loss of dignity: Experiences of older women living with incurable cancer at home. *Health Care for Women International, 41*(9), 1036–1058. https://doi-org.proxy.uwec.edu/10.1080/07399332.2020.1797035

Surico, D. (2014, March 1). *"Dining upgrades a la 'cart'"* McKnight's Long-Term Care News. https://www.mcknights.com/news/dining-upgrades-a-la-cart/

Tuominen, L., Leino-Kilpi, H., & Suhonen, R. (2016). Older people's experiences of their free will in nursing homes. *Nursing Ethics, 23*(1), 22–35. https://doi.org/10.1177/0969733014557119

Van Haitsma, K. (2019). *PELI-nursing home-MDS 3.0 section F-version 2.0. Preference based Living.* https://www.preferencebasedliving.com/for-practitioners/practitioner/assessment/peli-questionnaires/peli-nursing-home-mds-3-0-section-f-version-2-0/

Welford, C. M. (2012). Autonomy for older people in residential care: A selective lit-erature review. *International Journal of Older People Nursing, 7*(1), 65–69. https://doi.org/10.1111/j.1748-3743.2012.00311.x

Wood, D. (2016, August 24). *10 Ways to ensure respectful care of ICU patients.* American Mobile. https://www.americanmobile.com/nursezone/nursing-news/10-ways-to-ensure-respectful-care-of-icu-patients/

World Health Organization. (2011). *Palliative care for older people: Better practices.* World Health Organization. Retrieved from https://www.euro.who.int/__data/assets/pdf_file/0017/143153/e95052.pdf

World Health Organization. (2015). *World report on ageing and health.* World Health Organization. Retrieved from http://apps.who.int/iris/bitstream/handle/10665/186463/9789240694811_eng.pdf?sequence=1

Chapter 3
Relationships with Other Residents, Staff, and Family Members

Too often we underestimate the power of a touch, a smile, a kind word, a listening ear, an honest compliment or the smallest act of caring, all of which have the potential to turn a life around. – Leo Buscaglia

Abstract Relationships substantially impact resident quality of life. Research has indicated that residents value relationships with multiple constituencies. Resident-resident (peer) relationships, resident-staff relationships, and resident-family relationships are all explored. The value of peer relationships and how they contribute to a sense of belonging are examined, including resident preferences for and types of relationships, how proximity and peer activities or engagement opportunities help form such relationships, and how facilities can remove barriers and support residents' relationships with each other. Additionally, interpersonal relationships, including intimate or romantic interactions, that are either pre-established or newly formed after arrival at the care community, will be included. The importance of relationships between staff and residents is also described. Direct care staff often have the greatest potential to affect resident quality of life and, when residents cannot speak for themselves, may serve as accurate proxies for resident preferences. How these relationships support individualized care and emotional well-being is detailed, along with specific approaches and actions to promote such relationships. Finally, the promotion and facilitation of family member visits will be discussed, including options to do so virtually via technology when in-person visits are not feasible. Strategies for building connections with families are also highlighted, including the value of effective family councils.

Keywords Resident-resident (peer) relationships · Resident-staff relationships · Resident-family relationships · Romantic relationships · Individualized care · Emotional well-being · Quality of life · Engaging families · Family councils · Role of staff

Moving into a residential care community affects an individual's social network, often impacting existing relationships, but also offering opportunities to develop new ones. Long-term care recipients find meaning in relationships with fellow residents, family and friends, and staff within the care community. Residents rely on relationships of these three distinct types to support their psychosocial well-being in varied ways. Although moving into a long-term care community is likely to come with a period of adjustment, it also brings with it great potential to develop new social relationships and a sense of belonging, which can and do tend to develop over a short period of time (Scocco & Nassuato, 2017). Positive social relationships among long-term care recipients have been found to enhance well-being, life satisfaction, and quality of life (Bergland, 2007; Street, 2007; Roberts, 2018). Resident quality of life is impacted by physical and mental health (Naumann & Byrne, 2004), and while loneliness can threaten elderly people's physical and psychological well-being (Bianchetti et al., 2003), social engagement reduces the risk of negative physical and mental health outcomes (Drageset, 2004) and personal relationships play an important role in helping residents thrive (Bergland & Kirkevold, 2005; Bowers et al., 2001).

3.1 Peer Relationships

Peer relationships between and among residents foster a sense of belonging, purpose, achievement, and significance (Kang et al., 2020) and can promote a sense of feeling at home (Street, 2007). In fact, a move to residential care can decrease loneliness and increase the potential for developing new social relationships, especially for seniors who were increasingly isolated prior to the move.

Although peer relationships that develop in long-term care settings tend to have less intimacy than those established earlier in life (McKee et al., 1999), social relationships with care community peers may become more salient to their everyday well-being (Street, 2007). Residents get used to their new environment as time passes and many increase the number and quality of their relationships (Scocco & Nassuato, 2017), which positively influences their quality of life (Onunkwor et al., 2016). When care recipients are distanced from external, prior relationships, even casual friendships with fellow residents help fill in gaps and can result in improved well-being (Sandstrom, 2014).

As residents acclimate and adjust to new routines and community, the friendships they develop with peers promote a sense of familiarity, meaning, and belonging (Canham et al., 2017). Residents grow to care about each other and notice when their peers are gone—for example, when someone misses dinner or is hospitalized. Care recipients miss their friends and feel relief and happiness when they return; or if they themselves have been hospitalized, they may make comments like "It's nice to be home," upon returning, which emphasizes how positive peer relationships contribute to a resident's sense of community (Johs-Artisensi et al., 2020). Part of the "care" long-term care communities provide includes fostering an environment where residents' quality of life is enhanced by developing and maintaining friendships (Roberts & Bowers, 2015) through both structured and spontaneous socialization opportunities (Scocco & Nassuato, 2017).

Exhibit 3.1 Suggested Ideas for Resident Social Engagement when Infection Control Measures Require Physical Distancing
- Hallway soccer game played from doorways.
- Large muscle activities (e.g., exercise; yoga; tai chi; noodles, scarf, and stretchy band exercises) from doorways.
- Hallway joke hour: Residents take turns telling prepared and printed jokes.
- Remote control cars maneuvered in and out of the rooms.
- Singing in hallways/doorways between staff and residents.
- Church in the hall, or piped into resident rooms via television, radio, or other livestream methods.
- Fish or small animal tank on wheels.
- Bread machine in the halls for aroma and then deliver freshly baked bread to rooms for snacking.
- Daily bingo numbers given for an ongoing weekly game: every day at lunch residents receive 3 numbers until someone calls bingo.

Adapted from the National Certification Council for Activity Professionals' "Delivering the Social Model of Care During COVID 19 Restrictions".

Peer relationships within care communities were significantly tested when, during the COVID-19 pandemic, communities were forced to discontinue group activities, isolate residents in their rooms, and keep them apart from one another for their own safety. The stories of loneliness and isolation of residents were devastating, and the ramifications of such isolation are only beginning to be studied. Those who seemed to fare the best lived in care communities that found ways to support social relationships despite requirements to social distance, with examples of such measures provided in Exhibit 3.1. Stories abound of examples of safe social activities, such as overhead sound system trivia contests, hallway bingo, or ways for residents to eat alone at tables, yet be together in large dining spaces. Other facilities helped keep peers connected to each other through closed circuit televisions. One facility let residents participate in the shared experience of "virtual vacations," selecting a different country and streaming tourism documentaries, while another used a novel "cooking show" format featuring and connecting peers with each other (see Exhibit 3.2). These strategies were so beneficial that many care communities plan to continue these efforts into the future.

Exhibit 3.2 A Resident-Featured Cooking Show
One care facility got creative in thinking about ways to help keep care recipients connected with their peers. Activities staff came up with the idea of a "Cooking Show" that could be broadcast over the facility's closed circuit television system. They solicited participation from residents who were interested in being featured on the show to share a favorite recipe. The staff member interviewed the resident to learn more about why it was a favorite recipe and hear some stories about times they had eaten it or prepared it in the past. Staff then prepared a short video presentation that included pictures of the featured resident and dish, with an accompanying narrative about the history and memories assorted with the dish. Then they moved to a recorded demonstration of the staff member preparing the dish. Finally, once the show "aired" they used a cart to offer tasting samples of the dish to residents in their rooms.

This new socially distant activity quickly became a hit throughout the care community. Residents were able to "see" their peers, despite isolating, and learn more about them—their favorite food and special memories from their past lives. The featured residents also enjoyed the opportunity to be in the limelight. It became so popular that it remains a coveted activity, especially now that featured residents can be interviewed and participate "live" in the cooking demonstration.

3.1.1   Care Recipients Are Unique

As valuable as peer relationships can be for care recipients, they are not a homogenous group. The importance and value of peer relationships is dependent on multiple factors. For example, extroverted residents may need and crave social relationships, finding them energizing and recharging, whereas introverts may find them draining. For some, especially when just having been admitted to a care center, where significant energy is devoted solely toward maintaining activities of daily living, it may simply require too much cognitive bandwidth for the potential reward.

Some residents thrive despite having few peer relationships within the care center. They feel fulfilled enough by existing external relationships and don't deem intrafacility connections as important. Others may have fewer or less deep-level peer relationships than desired, perhaps finding it difficult to connect with those who have cognitive impairment or missing opportunities to socialize with those with whom they may share common interests. Additionally, other residents may be lacking well-being but don't see their lack of social relationships as playing a role in this. Because of this heterogeneity, it is important that caregivers are attuned and attentive to which residents are interested in increased peer socialization and which aren't, so they can intervene to assist those residents who want and would benefit from more or deeper peer relationships but are not able to meaningfully establish and maintain them on their own.

The level of social relationships among care community peers also varies. Many may lack the closeness of lifelong friends and family, but both acquaintanceships (where residents know each other's names or greet them at activities) and friendships (where special bonds exist beyond friendly greetings, mutual information is shared about families, or past lives or hobbies they enjoy are discussed (Roberts, 2018)), contribute to a sense of belonging.

3.1.2 How Residents Develop Peer Relationships

Although surface-level peer relationships may develop simply by sharing a space or participating in the same activity, for substantive friendships to occur, a higher level of engagement is necessary (Roberts, 2018). Initial bonds may be formed through group activities, dining together, or living on the same floor or neighborhood. But once meaningful social interactions are established, relationships can flourish as conversations ensue and residents seek out information about each other's past lives and current experiences. Care recipients may have a natural affinity for others who share common interests, as it gives them something to talk about and they can reminisce about past experiences together. Such peers often actively seek each other out to spend time together in organized activities or visiting on their own. Besides conversation and shared experiences, they may share snacks or token gifts or introduce one another to other residents or existing family and friends. Residents may also connect with peers altruistically, finding purpose in offering assistance to a peer who has physical limitations or working together as a team to complete a task, thus deriving a sense of achievement or significance. Some residents may advocate for those less able, to protect others' dignity or find ways to do small things to make fellow residents smile, facilitating others' sense of belonging (Kang et al., 2020) (Fig. 3.1).

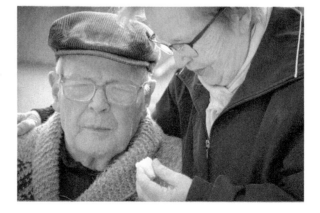

Fig. 3.1 A care center resident helps a friend to have a snack at an outdoor picnic. Sharing a treat or assisting a peer helps strengthen the bonds of peer relationships. Photo Credit: Gundula Vogel

3.1.3 Potential Barriers to Peer Relationships

Even when residents are interested in seeking out peer relationships, there can be institutional barriers within the care center. Among individuals with mobility challenges, pure physical proximity can be a potential barrier when options for socializing are limited to people seated near them during group activities. Even for more mobile residents, public spaces—whether quieter areas conducive to hearing conversations or busier places for those who enjoy keeping up with community happenings—may lack comfortable seating and a quiet enough ambiance conducive to socializing. Additionally, if a resident has a decline in health that necessitates a change of room or dining tables, lack of proximity to friends may cause established relationships to drift. Organizational processes or programming can also be a barrier. For example, mealtime service where those on special diets may not be served at the same time or the same table as others can interfere with peer socialization, as can a lack of social activity programs that match residents' previous or current interests. And, on occasion, regulations designed to protect care recipients' privacy can be frustrating when residents are unable to obtain information about a care community friend who is absent due to sickness or hospitalization (Kang et al., 2020).

A heterogenous clientele can also inadvertently impede peer relationships. Cognitively intact residents may be reluctant to interact with those who are cognitively impaired (Bergland, 2007) or those with aphasia or other communication disorders (Roberts, 2018). In some countries, like the United States, there is a trend toward nursing facilities serving both more traditional "long-stay" residents, as well as those staying for just a few days, weeks, or months, for rehabilitation and healing before returning home. Short-stay clientele often see themselves more as "patients" than residents and may lack interest in getting to know longer-term residents, sometimes even actively avoiding them to dodge the notion of becoming one someday. Simultaneously, long-term residents may be leery about investing energy into building relationships with people who will be leaving soon (Kang et al., 2020).

3.1.4 Facilitating Positive Peer Relationships

Offering a wide variety of organized activities ensures residents have ample choices to participate in leisure activities they enjoy and fit with their interests. However, simply ensuring a wide array of offerings is not sufficient; staff need to cultivate scenarios where positive and meaningful interactions can occur among residents. Sometimes a unique place for connections to occur is outside of routine activities and is associated with novel events like an outing, an activity held with a different peer group, or an event in a new location. This offers a chance to initiate conversations with new peers outside of typical routines or activities (Bergland, 2007).

Staff play an important role in how and whether social interactions or meaningful peer relationships develop. Staff should be supported, retained, and consistently scheduled so they have the opportunity to get to know residents well and what their interests and desires for social relationships are. Staff members, especially those providing direct care, need to have manageable workloads and should be trained and encouraged to bring residents together to facilitate conversations and build relationships. Examples of helpful conversation starters are presented in Exhibit 3.3. This can be done by introducing a general theme (e.g., current events, old characters or movies, favorite foods, traditional celebrations) and taking initiative to ask questions and encourage residents to share and connect by inviting them into the conversation. Staff can use information they know about residents to help make connections between those with shared interests or experiences. A good staff facilitator can make such conversations feel easy and enjoyable.

Exhibit 3.3 Discussion Starters for Facilitating Conversations Among Care Recipients

- Ask about their past.

    What is your favorite childhood memory?
    What did you and your friends do for fun when you were younger?
    What was the best lesson you learned?

- Ask about their present views.

    What is one piece of technology you think has changed the world for the better?
    How do you think the world has changed from when you were my age?
    What is something that made you happy this week?

- Ask them to look toward the future.

    What do you imagine (e.g., your grandchildren, a staff member) accomplishing in 10 years?
    How do you imagine the world will change in 10 years?
    How would you like to be remembered?

- Ask about their favorite things.

    What is your favorite type of show/movie/music?
    What do you like to do for fun and is it something we can do together?
    What is a new skill you would like to learn?

- Ask about accomplishments.

    What are you most proud of?
    How did your experience (e.g., in the military, as a teacher, during a particular time period) shape you?
    What lesson would you like to pass on to future generations?

Adapted from Griswald Home Care's "Senior Conversation Starters: Discussion Topics for Elderly Adults" (Rodriguez, 2019)

Residents tend to find personal conversations that go beyond small talk meaningful and enjoyable. Staff should be intentional about introducing or connecting residents to peers with similar hobbies, interests, personalities, and pasts. Introductions can occur in spaces like common areas, dining rooms, or shared bedrooms where residents will have both space and opportunity to communicate and explore the connection (Roberts, 2018). Staff may be able to engage some of the more extroverted residents to serve as peer connectors, even assigning them "official" positions such as greeters, matchmakers, or community ambassadors if such a role is welcome. This can boost their own sense of purpose and peers may be able to draw out some of the shy or less confident residents better than staff could.

Facilitating peer relationships among residents with cognitive impairment adds a challenge, as these residents tend to be more socially isolated (Roberts, 2018), but care communities are still responsible for finding ways to encourage such residents to be engaged, included, and feel like they belong. One suggestion is to have staff or volunteers spend time with resident pairs, rather than one-on-one visits, to help facilitate peer conversations and explore commonalities (Roberts, 2018). Dining is an event that naturally lends itself to being in close proximity and residents may especially enjoy the easiness of mealtime conversations if a staff member or volunteer shares the meal and takes the lead in facilitating (Bergland, 2007).

Unfortunately, peer relationships in long-term care settings, one certainty is that friendships will end when residents inevitably pass away. Peers of the departed may be well served if staff can offer them opportunities to grieve together, support each other, and share memories of their late friend (Fig. 3.2). Helpful practices to help residents process grief are shown in Exhibit 3.4. Staff may need to provide additional emotional support to grieving residents to assist them in processing their feelings, and once the resident is ready, staff can be intentional about re-engaging them in activities and introducing them to other residents who may one day become new friends.

Fig. 3.2 Unfortunately, loss of peers is a reality in long-term care centers, and cannot be avoided. Opportunities to memorialize peers are beneficial in helping residents to process grief and loss. Photo Credit: Kampus Production

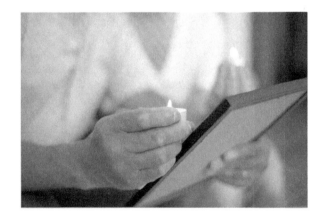

Exhibit 3.4 Supporting Residents Through Grief

In some care facilities, addressing care recipient deaths is avoided, seemingly in an effort to avoid upsetting other residents. However, many residents find that being given the opportunity to celebrate the lives of their friends aids them in their grieving process and allows for closure.

At Carlye Place in Georgia, when a resident death occurs, an electric candle is lit, the individual's obituary is shared, and a book is made available for fellow residents to write comments or share memories about their friend. They have even been considering establishing a "death café" where care community residents could gather in person to provide peer support as friends cope with death and loss, and hear stories of what others have experienced and how they got through it (Kaiser Health News, 2018).

Staff can also offer emotional support to grieving residents by giving them a chance to process their grief through conversation. After posing a question, then all the staff member needs to do is be open, interested, and respectful as they listen. Some possible conversation starters include:

- What kind of day has this been for you?
- What are some of the memories you are thinking about [name]?
- Who has been the most supportive to you, and how were they helpful?
- How has this been different than you thought it was going to be?
- What would you like people to know about your feelings right now?
- Are you still finding joy in going any of your usual activities?
- What do you want or need most right now?

Adapted from Cards and Conversations' "How Do You Talk with a Grieving Person?" (Chris, 2020).

3.2   Resident-Staff Relationships

Resident-staff relationships are multi-dimensional and include aspects such as friendship, therapeutic care, opportunities for engagement, communication, and autonomy (Scheffelaar et al., 2019). The relationships between staff and residents can impact care outcomes (Bowers et al., 2001) as well as resident quality of life and psychosocial well-being (McGilton, 2007). So, understanding the importance of these relationships, the role staff play in them, and how staff should be supported in these roles is critical to facilitating residents' emotional well-being. Post-admission, an initial adjustment to life in a long-term care community is to be expected. However, over time, as interactions with staff become more regular, residents and staff often develop relationships with feelings of attachment and affection which support residents' sense of home (Canham et al., 2017). This eases their adjustment and allows them to feel more comfortable, ultimately contributing to enhanced well-being and quality of life.

Positive resident-staff relationships lead to better life satisfaction for residents, specifically allowing residents to feel recognized, seen, and acknowledged as human beings (Scheffelaar et al., 2019). This builds connection and leads to a sense of belonging, which is vital to feeling at home later in life (Chaudhury & Rowles, 2005). For many residents, their relationships with staff significantly define their care community (Canham et al., 2017), and the more uncomfortable aspects of long-term care living, such as being dependent for care, a lack of privacy, or older building aesthetics can be overcome by this enhanced sense of community. It is not uncommon for administration to encourage staff to treat residents like family. Clearly defining expectations and supporting caregivers with both skills and time to develop relationships with residents will best support residents' emotional well-being.

3.2.1 How Resident-Staff Relationships Develop

As noted previously, residents may ascribe different levels of significance to relationships, including those with caregivers. Some residents have ample avenues outside of caregiver relationships that are meaningful and fulfilling and may be content to simply receive adequate assistance from skillful caregivers. Others may view and value caregiver relationships more generally and are content with caregivers considerately tending to their physical comfort and providing assistance with their activities of daily living—appreciating additional gestures of kindness and hospitality, but without need for specific personal friendships. However, some residents particularly value having close, personal, friendship-like relationships with their caregivers and may need those relationships to thrive (Bowers et al., 2001; Bergland & Kirkevold, 2005). Some care centers have utilized "buddy programs" or "guardian angel" programs as noted in Exhibit 3.5.

Exhibit 3.5 "Buddy Programs": Pairing Staff with Residents

Many care facilities have implemented programs, often titled "Buddy Programs" or "Guardian Angel Programs", where a staff member is paired with a resident to serve as a special friend and liaison. Often these partnerships are assigned at the time of admission and so the "buddy" can help offer additional support throughout the resident's adjustment to life in their new care community. Ideally, a relationship is built, and the "buddy" can continue to serve as a trusted staff member and friend to the resident throughout their time in the care center.

One such program exists at St. Ann's Community in New York. The role of the "buddy" is relatively informal, and buddies stop in for visits with their residents periodically—to check on them, have conversations, listen, or even assist them in starting a video chat with family members

(St. Ann's Community, 2020).

This aligns twofold with the philosophy of person-centered care. First, relative to the core principle of humaneness, person-centered care suggests that being valued by others is essential and promotes dignity (Eriksen et al., 2012). Secondly, all residents don't want their needs met in uniform ways, so cultivation of resident-staff relationships best supports individualized care and services for each person. Caregiver relationships are unique because, by definition, residents are dependent on staff for care. Several factors contribute to residents' emotional well-being—the resident, the human environment (caregivers), and the nonhuman environment (Haight, 2002). This suggests care communities must ensure staff are well-trained in delivering quality care and cultivating environments where relationships can flourish. Then staff, depending on the needs of individual residents, can identify the extent to which they should engage in further relationship development to maximize residents' emotional well-being and quality of life. An often-utilized resource for relationship building and culture change is the Pioneer Network, noted in Exhibit 3.6.

Exhibit 3.6 The Pioneer Network
The Pioneer Network is a leader in the United States for advancing culture change in long-term care communities—including helping elders' voices be heard, so they can direct their own care. They offer multiple free resources to support long-term care providers as they learn how to embrace care philosophies and put practices into place to advance culture change in their communities. A key goal of "culture change" is to help older adults feel "at home" wherever they live, which includes developing meaningful relationships among all those in their living environment. Pioneer Network has identified that a critical vehicle for facilitating resident—staff relationships is the care community's leadership supporting, nurturing, and empowering their staff in developing relationships with care recipients. Their website has a plethora of toolkits, exercises, and other resources to learn more about how to best support staff in developing relationships with residents (Pioneer Network, 2021).

3.2.2 Optimizing Resident-Staff Relationships

Caregivers offer more than just the provision of care, services, and supports. They offer a welcome interruption to the monotony of a resident's day-to-day life, stimulating conversation, comfort in times of grief or in the face of struggles, a link to connect residents to others or the outside world, and, most importantly, a sense of residents feeling at home. However, these are relationships that must grow over time, built on a foundation of trust and consistency from staff interactions over many shifts. Staff influence these relationships both through their approach—via their demeanor, and how they treat residents—as well as through their actions, by way of specific tasks or practices.

As the resident-staff relationship grows, the caregiver's presence, personality, and demeanor facilitate the development of trust. At their core, residents have a need to feel safe, and this is met by ensuring caregivers are knowledgeable and skillful in providing the individualized care and assistance each resident needs. As caregiver relationships commence, quality care provided with kindness can be the seed from which additional trust and confidence grows, through cyclical exchange. As trust grows, residents are likely to open up and share more, and as sharing occurs, trust further builds. The relationship becomes reciprocal, allowing caregivers to better learn residents' wishes and needs, which leads to them feeling seen, heard, acknowledged, and valued.

Residents respond best when they are treated with kindness and respect. Respect is demonstrated by caregivers in many ways, including being dependable, which engenders trust, and treating residents like equals rather than like children or ordering them around. As noted previously, autonomy is important to residents, so they value when caregivers help them exert their agency and make decisions together. For example, even though a resident may be dependent on assistance with dressing, their caregiver can still encourage their self-determination by asking them when they would like to get dressed and what they would like to wear. They can also help a resident feel known by anticipating their needs and offering assistance without burdening the resident to have to ask for help. These approaches help residents feel respected and it strengthens the trust and bond of their relationship.

Caregivers also build relationships by offering comfort and showing support. Listening to residents makes them feel heard. A perfect opportunity for resident-staff conversations arises while care tasks are being performed. These conversations with caregivers facilitate growth in resident-staff relationships without much extra effort—staff don't have to say much in response but can just listen to what residents are expressing. This demonstrates they are taking interest in the resident's life beyond the practical care they are providing, enhancing effectiveness by adding the additional element of emotional care (Fig. 3.3). Residents also appreciate being shown empathy. For example, when caregivers sense and acknowledge a resident's mood, it is validating and affirming. Finally, caregivers should explore ways to offer encouragement to residents. This can take many forms, such as offering empathy, emotional support, or advice, or empowering residents to make decisions. A final suggestion is using humor, although humor's reception is somewhat dependent on resident preference, which is why open communication is important. For some, having fun and laughing contributes to a good care relationship by lightening the mood, but others could perceive laughter as unprofessional or that a caregiver isn't taking them seriously.

Beyond how caregivers approach residents, there are other specific actions and practices that contribute to the quality of relationships. One approach is to use consistent staffing, as highlighted in Exhibit 3.7, which limits the number of caregivers a resident interacts with each day. The more opportunities residents and staff have to get to know one another, the easier it is to learn care recipients' individual needs and wants, which means all interactions and care can be personally tailored. A simple strategy is to have caregivers wear name badges with large letters,

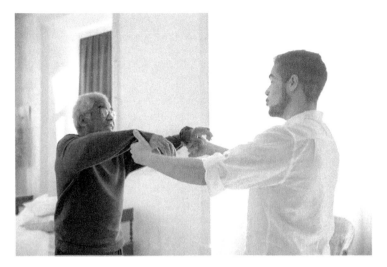

Fig. 3.3 A therapy assistant has a conversation with a resident while participating in restorative care. Such conversations lead to a strengthening of the resident-caregiver relationship. Photo Credit: Kampus Productions

that are easy-to-read, and have a picture of the caregiver. This is especially important if caregivers are wearing masks, so residents can feel a connection with the person behind the covering. Care tasks themselves can be delivered at the time of day and with the frequency the resident prefers. Care should be delivered such that the resident's privacy and dignity is preserved, which is especially important in shared or "semi-private" rooms or communal bathrooms. Caregivers can also affirm relationships by greeting residents by their preferred name, engaging them in conversations, making small talk, or offering them comfort with kind words to establish informal relationships beyond the provision of care. When residents share information about their family, or caregivers share about upcoming holiday plans or events, it offers a relationship that feels more like friendship than a purely transactional caregiving relationship. When caregivers engage in conversation or spend time with residents outside of prescribed activities, like dropping by during a meal or joining the resident in an activity, it heightens their bond. However, when informal relationships develop, caregivers should still strive to protect residents' privacy. When conversations occur specific to a resident's care needs, the discussions should become part of the care plan. However, if a resident shares a personal story, the caregiver should retain that confidence. Another area caregivers should be attuned to is physical contact. Physical contact occurs naturally in the provision of care and should be explained appropriately and performed gently during care tasks, but touch can also be a way to express emotional support (Fig. 3.4). For many people, a hand on the shoulder or a hug is comforting, although this may not be well received or appreciated by everyone. Knowing an individual's preferences helps caregivers understand which types of emotional support are most welcome.

Exhibit 3.7 Best Practices: Consistent Staff Assignment

What does consistent staff assignment mean?

Consistent assignment means residents see the same caregivers almost every time they are on duty. Residents are often more comfortable with caregivers who know and understand their personal preferences and needs. Consistent assignment is a key step in giving care that is centered on the resident. Consistent assignments build strong relationships between residents and staff, which are central to better care.

How does consistent staff assignment benefit residents?

- Residents don't have to repeatedly explain to new staff how to care for them or continually express their preferences.
- Residents feel more comfortable, especially with intimate aspects of care.
- Residents feel more secure with known caregivers.
- Residents and their families develop relationships with staff over time.

How does consistent staff assignment benefit caregivers?

- Caregivers know what each resident wants and needs, and can individualize care.
- Direct caregivers who work with the same residents most of the time may notice slight changes in health, preventing more serious problems.
- Caregivers are more likely to understand and better respond to the behaviors of residents with dementia, who often let others know what they want and need through their actions.
- Staff members better connect with residents they care for and are happier in their jobs.

How does consistent staff assignment benefit nursing homes?

- Staff get to know routines and develop deeper relationships with residents, making for a better workplace and a better home for residents.
- Caregiver absences are reduced and staff retention enhanced.

Adapted from Advancing Excellence in America's Nursing Homes' "Fast Facts: Consistent Assignment".

Having adequate staff with enough time to be able to perform not just care tasks, but also the extras—rapport building, emotional support, and informal friendships—are necessary for developing positive caregiver relationships. Many long-term care organizations have experienced staffing shortages which can lead to high turnover rates and a lack of consistency in caregivers, hampering the development of resident-staff relationships. One aspect of their job that caregivers value is the opportunity to develop relationships with their residents (Creapeau et al., 2022) so building an organizational culture that encourages resident-staff relationships by supporting staff with time and training can contribute to mutual benefits in a continuous positive

Fig. 3.4 A Caregiver expresses empathy to a resident through hand-holding. Sense of touch can be a powerful way to communicate care and affection. Photo Credit: Sabine van Erp

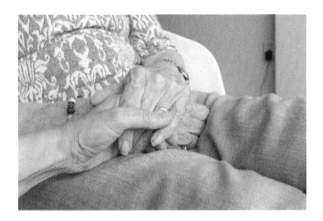

feedback loop. This allows residents and staff to mutually benefit from positive relationships, leading both parties to have greater satisfaction. When residents are calmer and happier, they are less irritated and agitated which improves their quality of life, as seen in Exhibit 3.8. It also leads to a less volatile environment which reduces stress on caregivers and increases their job satisfaction, making them more likely to stay, enhancing care continuity for residents, and further strengthening resident-staff relationships.

> **Exhibit 3.8 What Residents Value About Their Relationships with Staff**
> The relationships residents have with their caregivers is of utmost importance, as it was the most frequently mentioned factor from residents as to what enhances their quality of life. Residents value staff knowing who they are as people, treating them kindly, and being responsive to their needs and requests. Some of their comments included:
>
> *I have good relationships here and the aides are like my children. They know me so well, they are kind and just genuine with a heart.*
>
> *There's an excellent group of people running this place and they show complete interest in us.*
>
> *Every morning the aides knock on the door and tell us good morning. I really enjoy that they call my name as well. They really personalize the experience here.*
>
> *Adapted from "Qualitative Analyses of Nursing Home Residents' Quality of Life from Multiple Stakeholders' Perspectives" (Johs-Artisensi et al., 2020).*

Not only is it important to support and train staff in going beyond the care task portion of their job, but ideally the best staff to hire are caregivers who are open to developing personal relationships, are empathetic, have good communication skills, are trustworthy and dependable, and are sensitive to how individuals want to be treated and will act accordingly. Care organizations and staff should do everything possible to allow caregiver relationships to flourish. While deep caregiver relationships are not a necessary ingredient for every resident to have good quality of life, they are critical for some residents to thrive, especially those who lack other relationships or sources of meaning.

Although it is unlikely that positive resident-staff relationships have negative outcomes, one important caveat to consider, as staff develop deeper personal relationships with residents, is that those residents may eventually pass away. The risk of relationship is the risk of loss, and the grief associated with that. It is very important that care communities are attentive to and intentional in supporting their staff through grieving resident loss, as well. Some suggested practices to support staff members during the grieving process are displayed in Exhibit 3.9.

Exhibit 3.9 Policies and Practices to Support Caregivers Grieving the Loss of Their Residents

- Acknowledge grief reactions and the impact that they may have on staff as policies and procedures are developed.
- Offer confidential support groups, facilitated by mental health professionals, for staff to help them manage stress and cope with grief.
- Provide in-service education to prepare caregivers for managing the emotional experience of having a resident die.
- Share resources about grief and bereavement information and supports at workstations, break rooms, or other public staff spaces.
- Encourage family members of a resident who has passed to communicate directly with their caregivers, as many families may wish to thank caregivers directly and would love hearing caregivers share memories and stories of their loved one.

Adapted from Health Professions Press' "Supporting Staff in Long-Term Care as They Grieve the Deaths of Their Residents from COVID-19" (Kaplan, 2020)

3.3   Resident-Family Relationships

As they transition from home to the care community, residents are likely to miss face-to-face connections with loved ones. They may feel isolated with diminished social connections. This can lead to feelings of loneliness which occur when people lack a sense of belonging (Baumeister & Leary, 1995). Family relationships are an important factor that contributes to residents' quality of life (Johs-Artisensi et al., 2020). Although motivations may vary, family involvement and socioemotional support positively affect residents' overall physical and psychosocial well-being (Shier et al., 2013). Family visits are an antidote to resident isolation and loneliness and can counteract the consequences of social exclusion (Dewall, 2013). Beyond decreasing social isolation, involved family members who communicate and develop relationships with staff, help staff learn more about residents' preferences, interests, and past lives, and staff in turn can provide more individualized, person-centered care. When residents have positive social relationships and frequent visits with family and friends, the environment feels more homelike and comfortable, improving residents' psychological well-being (Miller, 2018).

3.3.1 Family Member Roles

Studies have identified numerous roles played by family members (Ryan & McKenna, 2014). The first is that of maintaining continuity of existing relationships and linking their loved one to the outside world. Regular engagement of residents by family members helps them maintain relationships, whether through face-to-face visits, video calls, telephone calls, letters, or sending small gifts. Those interactions keep the relationship dynamic and reassure the care recipient their loved ones are willing to prioritize time to support and maintain the relationship, and help the care recipient feel loved, connected, and important. On occasion, families may structure visits around events occurring within the care community, signaling to their loved one that they also want to participate in and belong to the care recipient's community. Through these communications and active engagements, friends and family can update loved ones about what is going on with family or in their former neighborhood, or take them on outings out of the building. This might include spending time outdoors, going for a walk, or bringing them to activities outside the nursing home, whether a trip to the store or restaurant, or home to visit family, friends, or pets (Fig. 3.5).

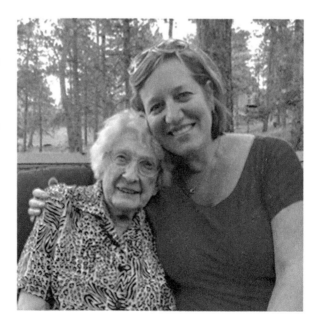

Fig. 3.5 Book co-author spending time outdoors during a visit with her grandmother who lives in an assisted living facility in Colorado. Maintaining relationships between residents and family members is instrumental for good quality of life. Photo credit: John Artisensi

Another family role is ensuring their loved one is receiving the best possible care and quality of life. Beyond decreasing social isolation, involved family members who communicate and develop relationships with staff can help staff learn more about residents' preferences, values, interests, and past lives, and staff in turn can provide more individualized, person-centered care. This is especially valuable for care recipients who have dementia and are not as able to communicate with staff independently. Another is for family to monitor and assist with their loved one's care. Family members can advocate to ensure both basic care needs, as well as the "little things," are being addressed by staff. On occasion family or close friends may even step in to provide such care directly. They can also be helpful in alerting staff to detect changes in residents' health status.

Finally, loved ones also may contribute to the broader care community by getting to know and interacting with other residents and their friends and relatives, staff, and leadership. This includes developing and maintaining various interpersonal social connections, perhaps organizing leisure activities, or advocating more broadly for changes that could enhance the quality of care and life for all residents.

One formal way in which families can embody the role of community contributor is through participation in family councils. These are comprised of self-selected family or friends who wish to protect and improve resident quality of life. Councils are an effective tool to help increase and enhance family inclusion (Baumbusch et al., 2020) by providing families information and education and facilitating communication between family members and staff. They offer an element of support and belonging among peer families who may have similar feelings and experiences. When families are involved in issues that affect their loved ones and other residents, their loved one may feel less isolated. Families can raise common concerns, have a voice in decision-making, and effect change by encouraging policy changes or enhancing residents' leisure time (Persson, 2008). Through fundraising, donations, and volunteer work, they can support activities programming, sponsor enrichment events, or facilitate new policies, such as increasing parking spaces for family, improving call light response times, and eliminating lost laundry (Curry et al., 2007). Thus, all residents can benefit from the engagement of family council activities, via community improvements, even if their personal family members are not participating. In some countries, formation of family councils is a right established in government regulations. Families are afforded the right to meet with other families in space provided by the facility, and although facility staff are only permitted to attend at the invitation of the council, the facility must designate a staff member to provide assistance, respond to requests, and take action on grievances raised or proposed recommendations.

3.3.2 Facilitating Resident-Family Relationships

The opportunity to be engaged in residents' daily lives, especially with the little things, is important to family members (Ryan & McKenna, 2014), so efforts to facilitate family involvement with residents are likely to be positively received (Hockley et al., 2021). This should begin at the time of admission, by welcoming and orienting families, including information and education about how the care community supports person-centered care, the role families play in that, and an invitation to them to participate in community life and support their loved ones in meaningful ways (Fig. 3.6). Facilities should encourage families to visit by making visitors feel welcome. This could include offering complimentary beverages or snacks, low-cost meals so families can dine with their loved ones, ample comfortable and private spaces for visits, and the ability to join in community activities with their loved ones. It is also important to reduce barriers, when possible, given some family members have transportation difficulties or other impediments, such as work schedules, chronic illness, or other obligations that make face-to-face visits difficult. Efforts should be made to use technology to support family connections with those unable to visit in person (Fig. 3.7). Effective practices for this include ensuring residents have access to internet service and devices that allow them to connect with

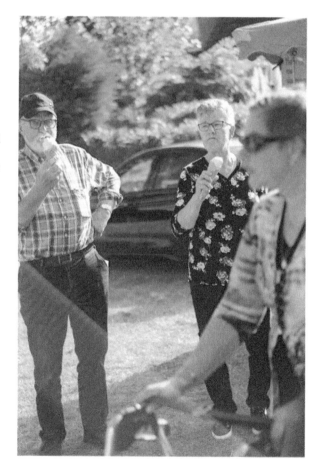

Fig. 3.6 A resident and family members enjoy an outdoor family carnival sponsored by the Family Council and hosted by the care community's Life Enrichment department. A strong Family Council offers families the opportunity to both be heard as well as advocate and effect quality improvements for members of the care community. Photo Credit: Sven Brandsma

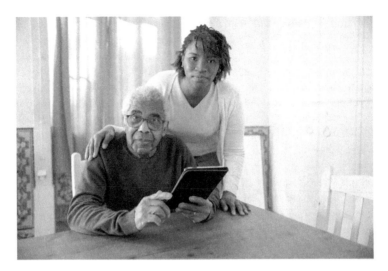

Fig. 3.7 A resident assistant helps a care recipient use a tablet to have a video visit with his family. This is beneficial in helping them to stay connected, even when physically apart—whether because of infection control protocols or simply because family live geographically far away. Photo Credit: Kampus Productions

family by video visit (or at least telephone) and providing adequate staff support to assist them in using technology, scheduling calls or video visits, and any assistance needed to conduct the call or video visit with family members. Technology-assisted visits may even strengthen the resident-staff-family triad when they require intentional staff member's involvement (Hockley et al., 2021). Facilities could even get creative about supporting occasional in-person visits by offering or subsidizing transportation or partnering with community groups that could assist families in overcoming geographic or transportation barriers, especially for residents whose face-to-face visits are infrequent.

Facilities should also seek to engage families in the care planning process. If the stage has been set at admission regarding a person-centered care environment, then families will understand the value of their engagement. Facilities should expect, encourage, and support staff in developing relationships with families, and opportunities for such engagement are highlighted in Exhibit 3.10. This allows staff to understand family members' perspectives and gain additional information about residents' interests and preferences, both informally through visits, as well as by including families in actual care planning meetings. Family members should be invited to such meetings in advance and offered options or flexibility in scheduling. If families are unable to be present in person, videoconferencing or conference call options should be made available. Families appreciate it when staff are receptive to issues they bring up, but they appreciate even more when staff are proactive. For example, if staff notice a resident feels sad or depressed, they can initiate contact with family members for a visit (in person or via technology). And, ultimately, when good quality care is provided, families are free to focus on socioemotional support of their loved one instead of worrying whether basic care needs are being met.

Exhibit 3.10 Opportunities to Engage Residents and Family
- Assign a leader to oversee facility efforts to evaluate and improve family engagement practices.
- Evaluate ways you currently listen to families (e.g., focus groups, learning circles, family councils), and identify ways to solicit input about families' expectations and how to best meet them.
- Conduct town hall meetings, "quality" care conferences, and individual meetings with residents and family members to focus on quality concerns and share efforts to improve quality.
- Communicate to families that resident quality of care and quality of life is a facility priority.
- Invite families to present at staff orientations and in-service programs.
- Explore the facility through the eyes of families by doing a "walk-about" with them.
- Include family members on teams that are developing quality improvement.
- Ask residents and families to help define what successful family engagement looks like.
- Provide updates on progress and monitoring during family council meetings.
- Develop a method to track families input and provide feedback on status of response to needs, concerns, or opportunities for improvement.
- Include families in team celebrations.
- Post stories of family engagement in facility newsletters and provide opportunities for family members to share their success stories with management and other staff.

Adapted from the Agency for Healthcare Research and Quality's "Resident and Family Engagement Checklist".

Staff partnerships are critical to promoting strong family relationships, so it is important staff are supported in doing so. With appropriate workloads, they will have time to devote to nurturing resident-family relationships. Staff also need education and training about the importance of their role in cultivating family relationships, how family members can support a culture of person-centered care, as well as how to use technology to support family visits or involvement in care conferences.

Care communities should offer opportunities for family engagement as described in the Activities and Religious Practices chapter, as it sends families the message that they are valued and instrumental in bringing joy to residents. Families may also benefit from educational or "support group" type programming, hosted at the facility. Offering workshops about dementia progression or support groups for family members of residents on hospice provides information, social connections with other families, and natural opportunities to visit loved ones before or after such sessions.

Especially evident during the COVID-19 pandemic, families like to have information and reassurance when they can't be present to see their loved one for themselves, and there are broader organizational strategies that can be employed to accomplish these aims (Hockley et al., 2021). Care communities should consider using periodic newsletters (printed or electronic) along with sharing other critical information or updates via mass messaging emails, texts, or telephone calls, leaving a weekly update on a voicemail message "hotline" that families can listen to, or even conducting interactive webinars for loved ones to join live or watch at their leisure (see Exhibit 3.11). Another communication strategy that arose from COVID-19 for many facilities is enhanced content on websites and an increased social media presence or established social media groups (e.g., Facebook, Instagram). This yielded both public relations benefits as care centers collectively promoted fun activities and interesting things their residents and staff were doing, so families (or even prospective care recipients) could see that residents were active, engaged, and smiling (Hockley et al., 2021). These methods show a different perspective than what is seen during one-on-one visits and also provided—especially on social media—the opportunity for external engagement as family members replied to posts or group texts and some even began to develop new relationships with other families. Family members seeing regular activity from their loved one's care community on their social media feeds also serves as an effective, regular reminder of their relationship with their loved one and may prompt them to nurture that relationship more frequently.

Exhibit 3.11 Care Community Family Webinars
During the COVID-19 pandemic, the Hebrew Home at Riverdale in New York utilized technology to host a weekly, interactive webinar for families, to keep families informed of the rapidly changing situation. About 100 families tuned in weekly to watch the presentation made by the community's interdisciplinary leadership team and ask questions.

Not only was it a valuable and efficient way to communicate information to families, but the ability to tune in, weekly, knowing that an update would be provided was comforting, and the ability for loved ones to participate allowed them to ask and have their questions answered as well as use the venue to express their gratitude and appreciation to the care team, which was an unexpected benefit.

Adapted from McKnight's Long-Term Care News', "Nursing home lessons from COVID-19: From family webinars to Zoom staff meetings" (Berger, 2020).

Families appreciate these enhanced communication strategies, but also want to feel they are being heard. Care communities must demonstrate they are listening to, identifying, and solving problems that arise. Avenues for families to bring concerns to leadership are important, whether via an open-door management approach, a suggestion box, or a more formal family council. Suggested methods for turning "complaints into compliments" can be found in Exhibit 3.12. Facilities should offer these various mechanisms and also have a process for communicating what is received and how it is being followed up on. Families want their concerns to be taken seriously and typically enjoy being partners in resolving issues and improving care. Family councils should consider ways to increase family involvement, such as scheduling meetings adjacent to education workshops or family-focused activities as well as considering times when families are most available. To increase inclusivity, councils should also consider hybrid options using technology (e.g., closed captioning, language translation) and invite those who are unable to attend in person. When family councils come up with suggestions, the facility social worker or local ombudsmen may be useful resources to consult for help in turning recommendations into new care community practices.

Exhibit 3.12 A Model Process for Handling Complaints

Step 1: Encourage Residents and Family Members to Share Concerns— Regularly ask residents and families to share concerns they may have, both informally (e.g., in the hallway during a visit) and formally (e.g., mailings, newsletter articles). Staff members' attentiveness and empathy, when approached with a concern, will set the tone for the interaction. They should stop what they are doing and give the resident or family member their full attention, maintain eye contact, and avoid negative body language.

*Step 2: Apologize and Take Information at Initial Contact—*Generally, staff should apologize for inconveniences and respond with understanding, recognition, and consolation to validate concern and distress. When possible, staff should address and resolve the complaint immediately. If the complaint persists, the facility's complaint procedure should be implemented.

*Step 3: Document the Problem—*All complaints should be documented on a readily available form noting the complainant's name and contact information, date, resident it relates to, the complaint/concern, expectations of complainant, and to whom it is being referred. It should include space to note the investigator's name, findings, actions taken, whether (and when) it is/was reportable to an outside agency, how findings are reported to complainant, notes, and whether the complainant was satisfied.

*Step 4: Designate a Staff Contact—*A single staff liaison should be designated as the family's contact during the resolution process for complaints not immediately resolved. For more serious concerns, letters should be sent,

(continued)

Exhibit 3.12 (continued)
including the staff liaison's name and contact information, and an estimated timeline for resolution.

Step 5: Gather the Facts—Investigations should include comprehensive interviews to understand the scope of the problem and identify underlying root causes. For policy-related complaints, collaborating with staff and gathering their suggestions for resolution helps build unity, but for more serious issues (e.g., theft, mistreatment), a more investigatory approach may be necessary.

Step 6: Formulate a Solution—Inform the resident/family as soon as a resolution has been determined. Beyond discussing the resolution, communication with the family or resident is another opportunity to reaffirm your commitment to resident satisfaction. If a policy has been changed for the benefit of all residents, include that in the conversation.

Step 7: Follow Up—Following up on all complaints is essential. The staff liaison should call the resident/family member to verify satisfaction with the resolution. For some issues a mutually agreed upon resolution may not be reached, so parties may need to respectfully disagree.

Adapted from the National Center for Assisted Living's "Turning Complaints into Compliments" (National Center for Assisted Living, 2005).

3.4 Romantic Resident Relationships

Romance, intimacy, and sexuality are all important to the human experience, and although many may view these as endeavors only for the young, studies increasingly contradict this assumption. Occasionally, committed or married couples enter long-term care communities together; however, at other times, residents may either be trying to maintain a relationship with an existing partner still residing in the community or engaging in a new relationship with a fellow resident. Whether a relationship is longstanding or novel, or with a fellow resident or a community-based partner, the personnel and policies of the care center also play an important role in supporting residents' autonomy to maintain or develop romantic relationships.

Romantic relationships are premised on intimacy—feelings of being important to one another, belonging, being valued, and being cared for (Panosh & Button, 2014)—and may also involve sexuality, which broadly encompasses thoughts, desires, attitudes, and behaviors, but may or may not include sexual intercourse (Macleod & McCabe, 2020). Although multiple biopsychosocial factors may influence sexual expression, especially among older adults (Delamater, 2012), and frequency, intensity, and possibility of sexual expression decline with age, older adults report even more fulfillment from intimacy and sexuality than their younger counterparts (Roelofs, 2018). A meaningful proportion of older adults, even though residing in care centers, remain or desire to remain sexually active (Wang et al., 2015; Lindau et al., 2007).

Quality romantic relationships in older age can positively influence health, well-being, and longevity (Stokes, 2017). Couples' primary partner relationships remain important to them as they age (Rahn et al., 2020), and for couples separated by one's admission to a care facility, although the adjustment to being separated can be distressing to both partners (Hunt, 2015), many continue to rely on each other for emotional support and intimacy even while living apart (Lewin, 2017). Additionally, many single older adults, including those residing long-term in a care community, long for the shared intimacy of a meaningful, partnered relationships (Malta & Farquharson, 2014).

3.4.1 Supporting Romantic Resident Relationships

Complex factors must sometimes be considered when supporting autonomy in romantic—and, particularly, sexual—relationships involving care recipients (see Exhibit 3.13). Romantic relationships that don't involve sexual contact can and should be supported similarly to any peer or family relationship. However, if sexual contact will be involved, additional concerns must be navigated. First, appropriate education to residents, family, and staff regarding residents' rights to participate in romantic relationships should be communicated, including assurance that all types of relationships (e.g., outside of marriage, interracial) and sexual identities (e.g., LGBT +) will be supported. Additionally, processes for assessing capacity and securing consent, practical support, and appropriate privacy for such activity to happen safely must occur. Ensuring a care recipient is capable of consent is best undertaken by their interdisciplinary care team. The care team can make certain the individual fully understands any associated health risks and their cognitive status can be assessed to confirm their ability to give consent. Within the care planning process, any measures that should be in place to ensure a safer encounter could also be addressed, such as providing education and protection from sexually transmitted diseases and mitigating falls risks. Facilities must also find a way to afford residents privacy. This may include procedures such as a "Do not Disturb" sign hung on the door to indicate that the resident and guest should not be interrupted by staff and serve as a reminder that staff should always be waiting to be invited in, even if they have knocked. Some facilities with shared resident rooms have established separate "intimacy rooms" so residents have privacy for intimate physical activity (Fig. 3.8). All staff should be educated about how the care center will support resident autonomy for consenting residents to engage in intimate relationships.

Exhibit 3.13 Steps for Accommodating Sexual Intimacy in Long-Term Care
Preparation

- Be aware of state statutes and case law on sexual consent.
- Draft institutional guidelines for management of resident sexual activity.
- Establish resources to support resident sexual activity:

  Resident sexuality consultation team.
  Offer an "intimacy room" for residents who do not have private rooms and appropriate signage.
  Educational materials for staff, families.
  Aids (e.g., lubricant, condoms).

- Hold staff training sessions.

Management

- Utilize a resident sexuality consultant.
- Conduct sexual consent capacity assessments.
- Develop an individualized care plan detailing how safety and privacy will be maintained.
- Hold staff support meetings.

Problem-solving resources

- Ethics committee consultation.
- Long-Term Care Ombudsman's Office.

Adapted from the American Medical Association Journal of Ethic's "Ethics and Intimate Sexual Activity in Long-Term Care" (Metzger, 2017).

Fig. 3.8 A couple, with one partner living in an assisted living facility, is afforded the privacy to maintain an intimate relationship. Intimacy, which can be achieved in myriad ways, is important to older adults' quality of life. Photo Credit: Brandon Robert

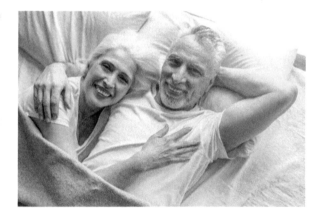

Occasionally, residents might make choices that others may disapprove of or feel uncomfortable about. For example, a resident might choose to be in intimate relationships with multiple people or with someone other than their spouse but, still, their autonomy should be respected. Family members may struggle with this emotionally, especially if their loved one has an existing relationship with a spouse or partner. It can even be difficult if a sexual relationship is not part of the equation, such as when a care recipient with dementia has a community-living spouse but develops an intimate relationship with a peer. They may no longer even recognize their spouse or realize they are hurting them, but they know they enjoy participating in activities and meals with their new special friend. It would only harm the care recipient's quality of life to be forcibly separated or prevented from spending time near their new special friend, but at the same time, the care recipient's spouse may need additional education and emotional support from staff to be able to eventually accept and support that peer relationship for the good of their loved one. Although the dynamics of resident romantic relationships can be complex, they can also be rewarding when staff are properly equipped to best support them.

3.5 Essential Influencers

Given the important impact relationships have on resident well-being, there are some key stakeholders who play especially important roles in fostering positive social or romantic relationships for care recipients.

3.5.1 Nursing and Direct Care Staff

Direct care staff spend the most time with residents and therefore have the most influential role in nurturing their social relationships with peers, family, and staff. Nursing staff set the stage for these new relationships as soon as the care recipient has been admitted—first supporting residents through their initial adjustment phase, and then cultivating a deeper relationship as time goes on. As they are intentional about developing personal relationships with residents and getting to know residents' personalities and preferences, this insight can be instrumental in individualizing the resident's care plan. As the caregiver's relationship with the resident grows, they will likely learn more about the resident's connection to their family, which may prompt them to be intentional about scheduling a video visit with them, if the resident has not been able to see them recently. If the caregiver is involved in the visit and begins to develop their own relationship with the family, this provides another avenue by which the caregiver can obtain additional information about the resident's past experiences and preferences, useful in further tailoring the care they provide to the resident. Staff can also use what they have come to know about the residents they care for to facilitate connections among and between the resident and their peers within the care community. Finally, nursing staff can also help residents considering sexual relations to think critically about any health or safety risks they are willing to assume, and assist them in making sure privacy needs for intimacy are met and balanced with any necessary supports and services to ensure safety.

3.5.2 Social Workers

A key role for social services staff is ensuring residents' psychosocial well-being, in part by ensuring their need for connection and social engagement is nurtured. Both at admission and at various ongoing points in time, social workers should cultivate an intimate understanding of residents' personalities, interests, and preferences. As they stay attuned to a resident's psychosocial status, they can guide others in the provision of emotional support and relationship development for residents. They are instrumental liaisons between residents, family members, and other care team members, as well as between family councils and facility leadership. Because social workers get to know care recipients individually, but also collectively, they may be able to assist Activities Directors in developing activities with the potential to bring like-minded residents together. Social workers are well-poised to support interpersonal relationships between all parties important to residents and may play varying roles with family members—sometimes serving as a connector or conduit, while other times, perhaps as an arbitrator, depending on the relationship dynamics at play. Social workers will also play a key role in ensuring a resident is capable of consenting to a physically intimate relationship, if such a relationship is something a resident desires.

3.5.3 Activities Director and Aides

Activities personnel are responsible for designing and conducting recreational and life enrichment opportunities, and they are probably the most instrumental staff in facilitating peer relationships. Directors should design programming options that align with residents' interests and leisure preferences, both for personal enjoyment, but also so they can have shared experiences with peers who have common interests and experiences. They must also periodically ensure that communitywide activities that encourage family participation are planned, promoted, and held, at times that will be convenient for family members to attend. Activities aides should be trained and skilled in facilitating conversations and relationship development among pairs or small groups of residents.

3.5.4 Dining Staff

The dining experience is an important vehicle for supporting relationship development. Dining staff should be intentional about seating friends nearby each other and those who seek to develop peer relationships with residents who have common interests. Dining staff should periodically check in with residents to understand whether their preference is to dine with similar tablemates regularly, and if so, whether they remain content dining with the same group. If residents prefer to have variety in where and with whom they dine, either to move away from relationships they have outgrown or in a desire to broaden their social network, this should be implemented. Serving staff should engage residents in conversations as they serve them, both to develop their own relationships with them as well as to spur resident conversations with each other. Food service directors or other dining staff should also occasionally dine with residents to further develop their own connections with care recipients and to facilitate peer conversations among tablemates.

3.5.5 Volunteers

Volunteers are an excellent resource to enhance relationship development for residents. Depending on the background, skills, and time availability of volunteers, they can cultivate their own one-on-one relationships with residents or assist by facilitating peer conversations and relationship development between resident pairs or small groups. Tech-savvy volunteers are a great resource to train and support staff and residents in setting up social media accounts, help them learn how to use devices to self-initiate video calls with family and friends, or assist with scheduling and resident support in conducting video visits. These opportunities can be an especially good way to integrate high school or college student volunteers into the care community.

References

Advancing Excellence in America's Nursing Homes. (n.d.). *Fast facts: Consistent assignment.* https://phinational.org/wp-content/uploads/2017/07/Consumer-Fact-Sheet-Consistent-Assignment.pdf

Agency for Healthcare Research and Quality. (2017). *Resident and family engagement checklist.* https://www.ahrq.gov/hai/quality/tools/cauti-ltc/modules/implementation/long-term-modules/module5/engage-checklist.html

Baumbusch, J., Yip, I., Koehn, S., Reid, R., & Gandhi, P. (2020). A survey of the characteristics and administrator perceptions of family councils in a western Canadian province. *Journal of Applied Gerontology, 41*(2), 363–370. https://doi.org/10.1177/0733464820961257

Baumeister, R., & Leary, M. (1995). The need to belog: Desire for interpersonal attachments as a fundamental human motivation. *Psychological Bulletin, 117*, 497–529.

Berger, L. (2020, July 7). *Nursing home lessons from COVID-19: From family webinars to zoom staff* meetings. McKnight's Long-Term Care News. https://www.mcknights.com/news/nursing-home-lessons-from-covid-19-from-family-webinars-to-zoom-staff-meetings/

Bergland, A. (2007). The significance of peer relationships to thriving in nursing homes. *Journal of Clinical Nursing, 17,* 1295–1302. https://doi.org/10.1111/j.1365-2702.2007.02069.x

Bergland, A., & Kirkevold, M. (2005). Resident–caregiver relationships and thrivingamong nursing home residents. *Research in Nursing & Health, 28,* 365–375. https://doi.org/10.1002/nur.20097

Bianchetti, A., Padovani, A., & Trabucchi, M. (2003). Outcomes of Alzheimer's disease treatment: The Italian CRONOS project. *International Journal of Geriatric Psychiatry, 18,* 87–88.

Bowers, B., Fibich, B., & Jacobson, N. (2001). Care-as-service, care-as-relating, care-as-comfort: Understanding nursing home residents' definitions of quality. *The Gerontologist, 41,* 539–545. https://doi.org/10.1093/geront/41.4.539

Canham, S., Battersby, L., Fang, M., Sixsmith, J., Woolrych, R., & Sixsmith, A. (2017). From familiar faces to family: Staff and resident relationships in long-term care. *Journal of Aging and Health, 29*(5), 842–857. https://doi.org/10.1177/0898264316645550

Chaudhury, H., & Rowles, G. D. (2005). Between the shores of recollection and imagination: Self, aging, and home. In G. D. (Ed.), *Home and identity in late life: International perspectives* (pp. 3–20). Springer.

Chris. (2020, September 14). How do you talk with a grieving person? *Cards & Conversation.* https://www.conversationcards.biz/How-do-you-talk-with-a-grieving-person_b_28.html?gclid=Cj0KCQjwiNSLBhCPARIsAKNS4_cXENNwAVRf-TYrrlVKH3ReSmHpKTwanv1uO9kZOU0bDdxmhl7ftXMaAsWvEALw_wcB

Creapeau, L., Johs-Artisensi, J., & Lauver, K. (2022). Leadership and staff perceptions on long-term care staffing challenges related to certified nursing assistant retention. *Journal of Nursing Administration, 52*(3), 146–153. https://doi.org/10.1097/NNA.0000000000001122

Curry, L., Walker, C., Hogstel, M., & Walker, M. (2007). A study of family councils in nursing homes. *Geriatric Nursing, 28*(4), 245–253.

Delamater, J. (2012). Sexual expression in later life: A review and synthesis. *The Journal of Sex Research, 49*(2–3), 125–141. https://doi.org/10.1080/00224499.2011.603168

Dewall, C. (2013). *The Oxford handbook of social exclusion.* Oxford University Press.

Drageset, J. (2004). The importance of activities of daily living and social contact for loneliness: A survey among residents in nursing homes. *Scandinavian Journal of Caring Sciences, 18,* 65–71.

Eriksen, K. Å., Sundfor, B., Karlsson, B., Raholm, M. B., & Arman, M. (2012). Recognition as a valued human being: Perspectives of mental health service users. *Nursing Ethics, 19*(3), 357–368. https://doi.org/10.1177/0969733011423293

Haight, B. B. (2002). Thriving: A life span theory. *Journal of Gerontological Nursing, 28*(3), 14–22. https://doi.org/10.3928/0098-9134-20020301-05

Hockley, J., Hafford-Letchfield, T., Noone, S., Mason, B., Jamieson, L., Iversholt, R., ... Tolson, D. (2021). COVID, communication and care homes: A staffs' perspective of supporting the emotional needs of familes. *Journal of Long Term Care, 2021,* 167–176. https://doi.org/10.31389/jltc.74

Hunt, B. (2015). *The emotional impact on elderly spouses who placed their loved ones in long-term care [dissertation on the internet].* Walden University. https://scholarworks.waldenu.edu/dissertations/1444/

Johs-Artisensi, L., Hansen, K., & Olson, D. (2020). Qualitative analyses of nursing home residents' quality of life from multiple stakeholders' perspectives. *Quality of Life Research, 29*(5), 1229–1238. https://doi.org/10.1007/s11136-019-02395-3

Kaiser Health News. (2018, September 4). *Dealing with death in long-term care.* U.S. News and World Report. https://www.usnews.com/news/healthiest-communities/articles/2018-09-04/dealing-with-death-in-long-term-care-facilities

Kaplan, M. (2020, June 19). *Supporting staff in long-term care as they grieve the deaths of their residents from COVID-19.* Health Professions Press Resource Center. https://blog.

healthpropress.com/2020/06/supporting-staff-in-long-term-careas-they-grieve-the-deaths-of-their-residents-from-covid-19/

Kang, B., Scales, K., McConnell, E., Song, Y., Lepore, M., & Corazzini, M. (2020). Nursing home residents' perspectives on their social relationships. *Journal of Clinical Nursing, 29*, 1162–1174. https://doi.org/10.1111/jocn.15174

Lewin, A. C. (2017). Health and relationship quality later in life: A comparison of living apart together (LAT), first marriages, remarriages, and cohabitation. *Journal of Family Issues, 38*(12), 1754–1774.

Lindau, S. T., Schumm, L. P., Laumann, E. O., Levinson, W., O'Muircheartaihg, C. A., & Waite, L. J. (2007). A study of sexuality and health among older adults in the United States. *New England Journal of Medicine, 357*, 762–774.

Macleod, A., & McCabe, M. P. (2020). Defining sexuality in later life: A systematic review. *Australian Journal on Ageing, 39*(Suppl. 1), 6–15. https://doi.org/10.1111/ajag.12741

Malta, S., & Farquharson, K. (2014). The initiation and progression of late-life romantic relationships. *Journal of Sociology, 50*(3), 237–251. https://doi.org/10.1177/1440783312442254

McGilton, K. S. (2007). Close care provider-resident relationships in long-term care environments. *Journal of Clinical Nursing, 16*, 2149–2157. https://doi.org/10.1111/j.1365-2702.2006.01636.x

McKee, K. J., Harrison, G., & Lee, K. (1999). Activity, friendships and wellbeing in residential settings for older people. *Aging and Mental Health, 3*, 142–152.

Metzger, E. (2017). Ethics and intimate sexual activity in long-term care. *American Medical Association Journal of Ethics, 19*(7), 640–648. https://doi.org/10.1001/journalofethics.2017.19.7.ecas1-1707

Miller, V. J. (2018). Investigating barriers to family visitation of nursing home residents: A systematic review. *Journal of Gerontologiocal Social Work, 62*, 261–278. https://doi.org/10.1080/01634372.2018.1544957

National Center for Assisted Living. (2005). *Turning complaints into compliments.* https://www.ahcancal.org/Assisted-Living/Provider-Resources/Documents/complaints_compliments.pdf

National Certification Council for Activity Professionals. (n.d.). *Delivering the social model of care during COVID 19 restrictions.* https://www.nccap.org/assets/docs/Delivery%20of%20Social%20Model%20of%20Care_Letter%20of%20Need%20%286%29.pdf

Naumann, V. J., & Byrne, G. (2004). WHOQOL-BREF as a measure of qual-ity of life in older patients with depression. *International Psychogeriatrics, 16*, 159–173.

Onunkwor, O., Al-Dubai, S. G., Arokiasamy, J., Yadav, H., Barua, A., & Shuaibu, H. (2016). A cross-sectional study on quality of life among the elderly in non-governmental organizations' elderly homes in Kuala Lumpur. *Health and Quality of Life Outcomes, 14*, 6. https://doi.org/10.1186/s12955-016-0408-8

Panosh & Button. (2014). *Recommendations for addressing resident relationships, board on aging and long term care – ombudsman program.* Retrieved from: https://ltcombudsman.org/uploads/files/issues/consent.pdf

Persson, D. (2008). Family councils in nursing facilities: Strategies for effective particiaption. *Journal of Gerontological Social Work, 50*(3–4), 51–63. https://doi.org/10.1300/J083v50n3_05

Pioneer Network. (2021). *We are here to help you every step of the way.* https://www.pioneernetwork.net/resource/

Rahn, A., Jones, T., Bennett, C., & Lykins, A. (2020). Baby boomers' attitudes to maintaining sexual and intimate relationships in long-term care. *Australian Journal on Ageing, 39*(Suppl. 1), 49–58.

Roberts, T. (2018). Nursing home resident relationship types: What supports close relationships with peers & staff? *Journal of Clinical Nursing, 27*, 4361–4372. https://doi.org/10.1111/jocn.14554

Roberts, T., & Bowers, B. (2015). How nursing home residents de-velop relationships with peers and staff: A grounded theory study. *International Journal of Nursing Studies, 52*(1), 57–67. https://doi.org/10.1016/j.ijnurstu.2014.07.008

Rodriguez, J. (2019, January 29). *Senior conversation starters: Discussion topics for elderly adults.* Griswald Home Care. https://www.griswoldhomecare.com/blog/2019/january/senior-conversation-starters-discussion-topics-f/

Roelofs, T. (2018). *Love, intimacy and sexuality in nursing home residents with dementia: An exploration from multiple perspectives.* DekoVerdivas. https://pure.uvt.nl/ws/portalfiles/portal/27445770/Roelofs_Love_05_09_2018.pdf

Ryan, A., & McKenna, H. (2014). It's the little things that count'. Families experience of roles, relationships and quality of care in rural nursing homes. *International Journal of Older People Nursing, 10,* 38–47. https://doi.org/10.1111/opn.12052

Sandstrom, G. M. (2014). Social interactions and well-be-ing: The surprising power of weak ties. *Personality and Social Psychology Bulletin, 40*(7), 910–922. https://doi.org/10.1177/0146167214529799

Scheffelaar, A., Hendriks, M., Bos, N., Luijkx, K., & van Dulmen, S. (2019). Determinants of the quality of care relationships in long-term care - a participatory study. *BMC Health Services Research, 19,* 1–14. https://doi.org/10.1186/s12913-019-4195-x

Scocco, P., & Nassuato, M. (2017). The role of social relationships among elderly community-dwelling and nursing-home residents:Findings from a qualityof life study. *Pychogeriatrics,* 231–237. https://doi.org/10.1111/psyg.12219

Shier, G., Ginsburg, M., Howell, J., Volland, P., & Golden, R. (2013). Strong social support services, such as transportation and help for caregivers, can lead to lower health care use and costs. *Health Addairs, 32*(3), 544–551. https://doi.org/10.1377/hlthaff.2012.0170

St. Ann's Community. (2020, March 17). *St. Ann's buddy program.* https://stannscommunity.com/buddy-program/

Stokes, J. E. (2017). Marital quality and loneliness in later life: A dyadic analysis of older married couples in Ireland. *Journal of Social and Personal Relationships, 34*(1), 114–135.

Street, D. B. (2007). The salience of social relationships forResident Well-being in assisted living. *Journal of Gerontology: Social Sciences, 62B*(2), S129–S134.

Wang, V., Depp, C. A., Ceglowski, J., Thompson, W. K., Rock, D., & Jeste, D. V. (2015). Sexual health and function in later life: A population based study of 606 older adults with a partner. *American Journal of Geriatric Pharmacotherapy, 23*(3), 227–233. https://doi.org/10.1016/j.jagp.2014.03.006

Chapter 4
Activities and Religious Practices

If a man is to live, he must be all alive, body, soul, mind, heart, spirit. – Thomas Merton

Abstract The content in this chapter primarily focuses on many of the psychosocial aspects that impact resident quality of life in long-term care settings through activities offered and religious or spiritual services provided. The number and variety of activities and programs scheduled for long-term care residents serve many important purposes related to optimal quality of life: increased physical activity, socialization with fellow residents and staff members, cognitive stimulation, community-building within and outside the care center, and more. Intrafacility activities and programs, as well as programming that incorporates external events, stakeholders, and organizations to engage residents with their surrounding community members are addressed. Activities designed or adapted for residents with cognitive impairments and for residents with physical impairments (e.g., residents who are ventilator-dependent, residents recovering from a stroke) are also covered, including adaptations that may permit residents with difficulties to be involved and socialize with other residents (e.g., virtual reality headsets, water aerobics for persons with mobility impairments). Lastly, the religious preferences and practices of residents in long-term care settings are addressed, including informal activities that may be scheduled as well as more formal religious services.

Keywords Activities · Religion · Spirituality · Events · Community · Physical activity · Water aerobics · Outdoor activities · Socialization · Cognitive stimulation · Programming · Music activities · Religious services · Meaningfulness · Purpose · Engagement · Individualization · Snoezelen rooms · Gaming systems · Virtual reality · Role of staff

One of the primary drivers of resident quality of life in long-term care settings are the activities and recreational events (i.e., programming) that are routinely scheduled. Individualized and engaging activities can provide a multitude of benefits: increased socialization, which enhances a sense of community through relationships and can

© The Author(s), under exclusive license to Springer Nature Switzerland AG 2022   77
J. L. Johs-Artisensi, K. E. Hansen, *Quality of Life and Well-Being for Residents in Long-Term Care Communities*, Human Well-Being Research and Policy Making,
https://doi.org/10.1007/978-3-031-04695-7_4

decrease feelings of depression; physical activity, to augment or complement any therapy regimens; and an ability to better and more fully acclimate to a new "home" upon admission to a care center. Activities in many long-term care communities often include religious or spiritual events to more comprehensively meet residents' needs, whether formally scheduled religious services like those residents may have experienced when living in their former home or informal activities, such as smaller gatherings for studying religious texts. And, even when experiencing physical or cognitive impairments, most residents are still able to participate in appropriately modified activities and receive enjoyment from engagement, as well as noted physiological and psychosocial benefits.

4.1 Psychosocial Benefits of Activities

The social benefit of activities cannot be emphasized enough for its impact on residents' mental health and psychosocial well-being. When programmed events are tailored to the activities residents enjoyed prior to admission to the care center, there is heightened engagement and enjoyment that aids residents in staving off depressive thoughts, anxiety, or emotional stress from the transition to a residential care setting. If residents are feeling depressed, they may disengage from activities, which has the effect of exacerbating depressive symptoms and increasing feelings of loneliness as they become further isolated and disengaged from their peers. However, the converse is also true, as resident participation in activities can help to pull them out of this spiral and reduce depressive symptoms. A helpful list of items for care centers to assess their programming is found in Exhibit 4.1. Additionally, residents spending the majority of time in their room may perseverate on negative feelings rather than looking ahead to an activity they enjoy or socializing with other residents and developing relationships further.

Exhibit 4.1 Checklist for Care Centers to Assess Emotional Health Promotion and Goals for a Whole Population Approach to Wellness Facility Assessment

- Do you have a variety of activities that promote intellectual, creative, spiritual, and physical well-being?
- Do you have programs and support services for residents that help them cope with loss?
- Have your staff received training on the value of engaging residents in intellectual, social, physical, and creative activities?
- Do you have programs that are designed to promote social networks and community building among your residents?

(continued)

Exhibit 4.1 (continued)

- Are you familiar with initiatives recommending improvements in the social and physical environment of a senior living community to increase resident well-being and satisfaction?
- Does your staff know how to screen for and identify the symptoms of depression and encourage residents to participate in activities?

Facility Goals for the Whole Population

- Activities: Residents have access to activities that promote their emotional health and well-being.
- Social networks: Participation in facility events and programming leads to established and enhanced social networks among residents.
- Staff training: Staff receive training and support for their roles in promoting activity promotion and emotional health of all residents, whether serving in a direct care staff role or not.

Adapted from the United States Department of Health and Human Services, Substance Abuse and Mental Health Services Administration's "A Guide to Promoting Emotional Health and Preventing Suicide in Senior Living Communities (SAMHSA, 2011).

Obviously, residents in care centers have either retired from their professional careers or are no longer busy with more traditional intra-community activities, such as going to work, raising a family, or engaging in various events (e.g., church, going to the grocery store, shopping). Programming and events in care centers can be a way to fill this "void" and provide needed structure each day. To this point, in studying residents in Malaysian nursing homes, Ibrahim and Dahlan (2015) discussed how activities tailored to residents' occupational life prior to admission would facilitate better sense of purpose. Exhibit 4.2 provides some sample questions to ask residents upon admission to aid in tailoring activities. This can aid residents in achieving a higher quality of life and has also been shown to prevent functional decline (Menec, 2003).

Exhibit 4.2 Sample Questions for an Admissions Questionnaire with Residents to Learn About Their Life Story

- Do you have a nickname?
- Where were you born?
- Where did you grow up? Could you describe the house you lived in?
- What time do you like to get up in the morning? Describe your routine after waking up.
- Do you enjoy taking naps?
- What are your typical routines in the afternoon and evening?

(continued)

Exhibit 4.2 (continued)
- Where did you go to school? What was your major if you went to college?
- What was your first paid job? Did you enjoy it?
- What was your favorite job? Why did you enjoy it so much?
- What are your hobbies and interests?
- Do you have any favorite movies or books? If so, which ones?
- What kind of music do you enjoy?
- Did you travel anywhere meaningful to you? If so, where were some of your favorite destination(s)?
- What have been some special events in your life?
- What's your favorite time of the year?
- Do you like pets? Are you allergic to any pets?
- Do you prefer solitary activities, small groups, or large groups?
- Did you attend a place of worship? Did you have a role in any of the services there?
- What makes you feel happy? What makes you feel sad? What helps alleviate this feeling?

Adapted from Crisis Prevention Institute's "Life Story Questionnaire" (CPI Dementia Care Specialists, 2015).

Some surveys—designed to evaluate resident quality of life—have also assessed whether activities are "meaningful" or not, with residents and family members highly valuing meaningful activities as important to resident quality of life (e.g., Tellis-Nayak et al., 2010). Activities and programming that provide meaning and purpose to residents can aid in the development of a new identity for residents and bolster self-esteem by replacing lost roles, under notions of role theory in gerontology, leading to better overall resident health (Krause et al., 1992). Recent evidence also indicates that residents' perceptions of and participation in activities, especially when it aids in building a sense of community within the care center, contribute to a feeling of purpose and vastly improve quality of life (Johs-Artisensi et al., 2020). Even residents with cognitive impairment (i.e., dementia) can reap the benefits from thoughtful activities, such as increased happiness, better alertness, less boredom, improved self-performance of activities of daily living (ADLs), and improved overall quality of life (Cohen-Mansfield et al., 2009). Some care communities have utilized information gathering processes upon a resident's initial admission to glean historical events in the resident's life to incorporate in planned activities and better achieve meaning and purpose via programming and events.

Activities also play an important role in giving residents of long-term care communities dignity. In evaluating nursing homes in Denmark, Norway, and Sweden, Slettebø et al. (2017) advocated for the need to identify residents' preferences related to participation in activities and the designing of events themselves. They suggested that activities tailored to residents' unique needs could "promote physical activity, social stimulation, and a sense of identity that may slow age-related decline"

(Slettebø et al., 2017). A French study of nursing home residents' activities noted that when a wide range of programming and activities providing "entertainment, relaxation, vitality, and stimulation to participate" were offered, residents had more enjoyment in their new care setting and adapted more readily to the environment (Altintas et al., 2017). Additionally, residents who engage in activities are more likely to thrive in their new home at the care center, meaning residents are experiencing optimal or beneficial well-being in relation to the environment around them (Björk et al., 2017).

4.2 Frequency and Variety of Activities

Many care communities have increased their focus in recent years on regular, frequent activities and events to boost metrics of customer (i.e., resident) satisfaction and to entice potential residents to join their care communities. Historically, however, it has not been uncommon for care centers to only schedule activities during limited amounts of time each day (e.g., Cohen-Mansfield et al., 1992, 2009). Often, the quality and quantity of events can be a differential advantage a facility can leverage in the marketplace over their competition to attract prospective residents. For communities with more active residents, such as assisted living centers, activities can play an even more prominent role for residents and can even be directed or led by residents in some cases. Numerous care centers have created monthly calendars of events (see sample ideas in Exhibit 4.3) to distribute to residents—and to families, for their participation as well—to stimulate engagement and promote positive psychosocial effects. Calendars provide a way for residents to plan which events they might like to attend and provide a reminder to staff members to think about potential holidays each month to inspire scheduled events. Additionally, cultural events important to various residents in the care center can be thoughtfully incorporated to ensure all members feel welcome and respected within the scheduled events. Instead of paper calendars distributed to residents, some care centers have utilized a closed-circuit television channel to display upcoming events in residents' rooms. While staples of traditional activities and programming in care centers—such as playing bingo, chess and checkers, or various card games in groups—may always be popular, facilities have developed a multitude of creative alternatives to give residents choice and variety each week to keep engagement high and residents interested.

> **Exhibit 4.3 Weekly Schedule of Calendar Ideas for Care Centers**
> **Monday**
>
> - 9:30 am: Bible Study in the Chapel
> - 11:00 am: Chair Yoga in the Community Center

(continued)

Exhibit 4.3 (continued)
- 1:30 pm: Bingo in the Activity Hall
- 3:00 pm: Book Club and Discussion in the Lounge

Tuesday

- 9:30 am: Checkers Olympics in the Lounge
- 11:00 am: Finger Painting with Elementary School Students in the Community Center
- 1:30 pm: Ice Cream Social in the Activity Hall
- 3:00 pm: Movie Matinee in the Community Center

Wednesday

- 9:30 am: Beautify with Manicures and Pedicures
- 11:00 am: Water Aerobics with Sam
- 1:30 pm: Buck Euchre Tournament in the Lounge
- 3:00 pm: Tai Chi in the Activity Hall

Thursday

- 9:30 am: Bible Study in the Chapel
- 11:00 am: Drum Circle with the "Lion King"
- 1:30 pm: Mindfulness and Meditation in the Lounge
- 3:00 pm: Wine and Art Event in the Activity Hall

Friday

- 9:30 am: Bean Bag Toss Tournament in the Community Center
- 11:00 am: Music and Memory Time in the Lounge
- 1:30 pm: Piano Concerto with Bill and Susan
- 3:00 pm: Cake and Celebration of October Birthdays in the Activity Hall

It has become rather appealing in many care centers to incorporate music into the activities that are scheduled. Sample questions to ask residents to aid in creating personalized playlists are found in Exhibit 4.4. This could include activities where the residents themselves play music or sing, or where local performers are invited to the care community to perform. Some care centers have even asked staff members to perform, if so inclined, to engage further with residents, like a talented housekeeper playing the piano during the day or during a meal. Such activities often utilize music that is from an earlier time in the residents' lives to evoke pleasant memories and can be delivered in various ways, such as online streaming services, iPods, or CD players that can utilize customized playlists for individual residents (e.g., Music and Memory, 2021). Some facilities have implemented drum circles, where residents use a variety of percussion instruments to play music and engage in activity that has both physical and emotional or psychosocial benefits (e.g., relaxation for residents, mindfulness benefits) (Golden Carers, 2021). Many care centers also utilize music around holidays and sometimes encourage intergenerational programming, such as having a local elementary school choir sing carols for residents near Christmas, which provides entertainment and socialization alike for residents and the children.

Exhibit 4.4 Questions to Ask Care Center Residents to Build a Personalized Music Playlist

- What types of music did you listen to when you were young and as you were growing up?
- Were you involved with music during any religious services growing up or during your adult life? Did you have any favorite hymns or songs?
- Are you a fan of any particular Broadway musicals or songs from musicals? Which are your favorite(s)?
- Did you have any records, tapes, or CDs with your favorite songs that you played often?
- Do you have a favorite artist that you listened to regularly? Or perhaps a famous band or orchestra? Who are they?
- Can you sing or hum the melody of any of your favorite songs?
- Do you have any songs from significant life events (e.g., proms, weddings, birthdays) that you really enjoy?

Adapted from Music and Memory's "How to Create a Personalized Playlist for Your Loved One at Home" (2012).

Physical activity should also be thoughtfully incorporated into activities, based on residents' abilities, and is another facet of activities and programming to engage residents. While, conceptually, physical therapy, occupational therapy, and speech-language therapy may occur separately, there are numerous activities that can build in a physical component to get residents up, mobile, and exercising to promote overall health (Fig. 4.1). One program that has gained popularity is chair yoga, where residents can engage in yoga practices while remaining seated. Other fitness activities, similar to the "Sit and Be Fit" program (Sit and Be Fit, 2021), focus on upper body exercises the resident can perform while seated or movement programs where residents use chairs to aid in balance (Daily Caring, 2021). Additionally, other activities incorporating even more physical activity can be planned and may include walks around the care center (with assistance, as needed), dancing classes or special events (e.g., a "senior prom"), or gardening. Gardening, for many residents, is a familiar and enjoyable activity that can thoughtfully incorporate moderate physical activity into a fun event. In providing gardening activities, care centers can also provide necessary tools (e.g., gloves, spades, watering cans) and other supplies (e.g., seeds to plant, soil, fertilizer). Even more ideal, any vegetables or fruit grown in the resident gardens can be used in the care center for meals to enhance resident satisfaction with the dining experience.

For care centers that have a pool or are in close proximity to a community center with one, water aerobics are often perceived by residents as a fun activity that

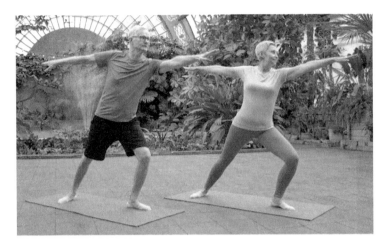

Fig. 4.1 Various complementary and alternative medicine practices have become integrated over time into activities for residents in care centers, including yoga or tai-chi programming. These activities can promote strength building and balance training for residents who may be at risk for falling, but also have been found to be enjoyable by many residents. Additionally, such activities can be modified for residents who may have mobility issues (e.g., chair yoga for residents who may have balance issues or lower-extremity weakness). Photo Credit: Marcus Aurelius

reduces stress on joints while providing natural resistance in the water to do some exercises. Activities that build in a physical exercise component and which promote resident safety can aid in reducing pain, building strength in older adults experiencing sarcopenia, promoting better sleep at night, improving mood, decreasing stress, reducing fall risks, and even minimizing agitation for residents with cognitive impairments (Harvard Health, 2019) (Fig. 4.2).

Care centers have also invested in gaming systems (e.g., Nintendo Wii, Microsoft Xbox) that have devices to capture a player's movements and simulate real sports or games to engage residents physically. For example, the Nintendo Wii controller is used in a way as one might swing a tennis racket or roll a bowling ball, helping residents develop strength and improve mobility (MyElder, 2021). Use of gaming devices also promotes additional intergenerational programming with family as an activity that a grandparent can enjoy with their grandchild during a visit to the care center. Other facilities have partnered with start-up companies or nonprofit organizations focusing on technology use for older adults (e.g., Thrive Center, 2021) to utilize virtual reality headsets (e.g., AppliedVR, MyndVR). These devices can be used safely in a number of ways to enhance resident quality of life, including "virtual vacations" where the resident never has to leave the building.

There are also numerous activities that can be scheduled which promote education and cognitive stimulation, an added benefit beyond physical activity (Fig. 4.3). As noted, activities tailored to residents' specific preferences can enhance functional capacity and reduce age-related declines (Slettebø et al., 2017). Cognitive stimulation can engage residents while simultaneously challenging the brain to delay normal age-related changes and potentially improve functioning for those residents with

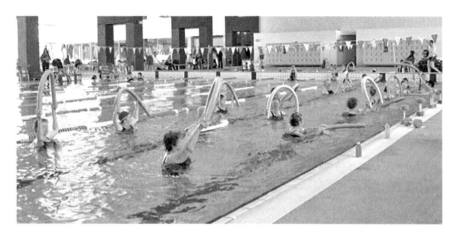

Fig. 4.2 Water aerobics onsite at the care center or at a nearby pool (e.g., YMCA, community pools near the care center) can be an enjoyable activity for residents—including residents with physical impairments or mobility issues—that promotes physical activity without pain or undue stress on joints. Beyond structured activities themselves, many residents enjoy leisurely swimming and being in the water, which is another way to promote socialization and have variety in the activities routinely scheduled. Photo Credit: Photo by www.localfitness.com.au

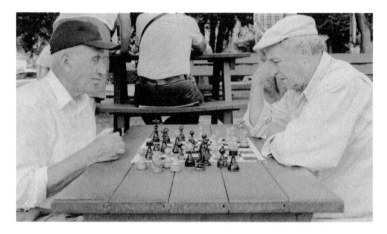

Fig. 4.3 Older residents engaging in activities that promote cognitive stimulation—such as chess, which requires strategy against one's opponent—can be easily incorporated into many activity schedules in care centers. There are numerous app-based games, in addition to more traditional board or card games, that older adults can play on tablet devices, smartphones, or computers which can surreptitiously embed cognitive training in a game the older adult resident enjoys. Photo Credit: Vlad Sarguin

dementia. Some care centers have brought in local artists to do a painting class with residents, while others have invited chefs to conduct a cooking class for residents, crafting a recipe with ingredients brought for the event.

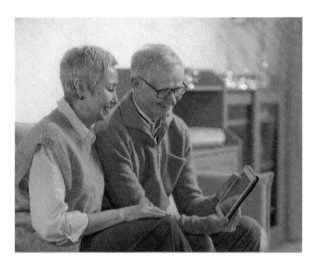

Fig. 4.4 Older adults have increasingly grown familiar with using technology to play games, take college courses later in life, and to video chat with family and friends near and far (e.g., Zoom, Facebook Messenger, Skype). Especially during the COVID-19 pandemic, tablet devices and smartphones were extraordinarily helpful to keep family members connected when in-person visits were not possible. Devices can even be used intrafacility to connect residents to one another and engage in group activities (e.g., card games played together from an app, video calls to fellow residents that are quarantined in room). Photo Credit: Marcus Aurelius

Some care centers have pursued grant funding or invested in tablet devices (e.g., iPad, Surface) to provide electronic games or activities to residents for those who may prefer a more solitary option (Fig. 4.4). Tablet-based activities, such as Lumosity (2021), can covertly embed cognitive training so older adults may not even realize their enjoyable game is simultaneously improving memory, cognitive speed of processing, executive function, and attention. Other activities possible through technology include networking and video visits with family members. One such program is called "It's Never Too Late" (IN2L, 2021), which allows a resident to create their own profile with content and applications tailored to their preferences, including games played individually or in a group with other residents at the care center. With increased technology available, other activities have included access to college courses for residents who may wish to expand their horizons or previously were unable to attend a university. Some college campuses make programming available virtually for adults age 65 and older, including those who may live in a care community, and this can be offered to residents as part of programming each month (e.g., Bellarmine University Veritas Society, 2021).

One subset of residents may benefit from even more targeted activities and events in care centers, namely, veterans. In the United States, the Department of Veterans Affairs operates nursing homes called Community Living Centers for former military service members. Such care centers often have special activities around federal holidays, such as Memorial Day and Veterans Day, to honor the prior service of residents and their family members. Other communities that have service and

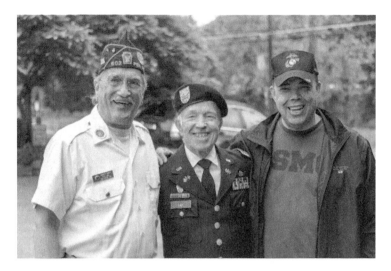

Fig. 4.5 During several holidays in the United States set aside for veterans—namely Memorial Day in May and Veterans Day in November—many care centers hold special events to recognize the former military service of their residents. This is even more so the case with nursing homes under the United States Department of Veterans Affairs—now called "Community Living Centers"—that incorporate many events throughout the year to recognize their members' service (e.g., a Veterans Ball held each year to incorporate spouses and members of the community that may not live at the Community Living Center with a spouse). Photo Credit: Craig Adderley

non-service member residents will often hold similar activities and may partner with local Veterans of Foreign Wars (VFW) or American Legion groups in the community, providing further opportunity for residents to mingle with broader community members (Fig. 4.5). Some care communities also partner with national organizations, such as Honor Flight (2021), to take resident veterans to the nation's capital and see the memorials and monuments related to their military service.

While many activities are planned and held within the care center, there is also great value in partnering with the surrounding local community to hold events at the facility or to get residents out and about around town. The National Consumer Voice for Quality Long-Term Care (2011) created a tip sheet that includes helpful ideas for building community involvement while actively incorporating residents into the process, such as holding a poster and crafts fair at the care center, developing a speaker series, hosting or sponsoring an education program at the facility, and creating a "community advisory panel" that residents can actively participate in for civic engagement. Some care centers have also served as polling places for state and federal elections, providing enhanced voting access for residents and serving as another event to invite community members into the care center.

During periods of social isolation, local community members can be a source of engagement, activities, and support for residents in care centers. LeadingAge, a national organization representing nonprofit care centers in the United States, highlighted various activities organized by community members for residents (see

Exhibit 4.5), such as partnering with a local Girl Scout troop to make care packages, creating videos for residents in partnership with a local performing arts school, holding virtual fitness classes, going on "virtual vacations" through viewing documentaries, and having retired clergy come for spiritual activities and visits (LeadingAge, 2021). Additionally, service trips to the community may be an ideal activity for older adults who may want to give back in their retirement years. Some care centers have scheduled trips where older adult residents go to a public library to read to children or volunteer at a shelter or soup kitchen for individuals who are homeless. Outdoor activities, even if close to the facility, are also incorporated into many recreational activities schedules, including wheelchair walks through the community or a trip to a local lake for a fishing outing, with staff members assisting. These trips can also easily incorporate family members or community-dwelling friends of the residents to enhance social engagement and enjoyment by the residents who participate.

Exhibit 4.5 Engaging Care Center Residents During Periods of Social Isolation or Quarantine
- Working with high school or college students to create care packages that have games, puzzles, and crosswords for in-room activities.
- Making a music video with residents, filmed from afar in their rooms, to do "doorway dances" and share with families, fellow residents, and community members.
- Holding virtual fitness classes through closed-circuit television channels in the care center for residents to remain physically active in their rooms.
- Scheduling resident-led activities for those in their rooms—through use of technology—such as Qigong, tai-chi, comedy hours, karaoke sessions, and Bingo.
- Creating virtual vacations via headsets showing the desired travel destination or looking online using computers to imitate the travel experience.
- Using tablet devices and computers to have regular video chats with family, friends, and community members that must remain apart.
- When permitted and feasible, holding outdoor activities on the care center campus for yoga, meditation, and stress reduction while staying physically distanced.

Adapted from LeadingAge member communities' "Resident Engagement During Social Isolation" stories (2021).

Care communities should offer family engagement activities and educational programming to promote their involvement with residents. Planning activities thoughtfully so families can attend and interact with loved ones, other residents, and staff can indeed be challenging, especially because families are most likely to be available during evenings or weekends, which is typically not when leadership is as readily available. However, the benefits of larger scale activities, with intergenerational attendees and opportunities for families to mingle and meet other families, especially in the context of a fun activity onsite or holiday-themed event, send the message to families that they are valued, and can bring joy to many residents in a care center. The benefits of incorporating intergenerational programming into care centers are highlighted in Exhibit 4.6.

Exhibit 4.6 Benefits of Scheduling Activities that are Intergenerational in Care Centers
Benefits to Older Adult Residents

- Reducing feelings of social isolation for older adults.
- Increased activity leads to approximately 20% more calories burned each week.
- Increased physical mobility (e.g., fewer falls, reduced reliance on assistive devices such as canes or walkers).
- Heightened performance on memory exams.
- Learning of new technology and communication skills.
- Improved outlook on aging and increased sense of purpose.

Benefits to Younger People

- Less likely to start using illegal drugs.
- Potential for alcohol abuse is decreased, as the likelihood to start drinking declines.
- Increased trust and communication with parents.
- Less likely to experience depressive symptoms.

Adapted from the Elder Care Alliance's "The Benefits of Intergenerational Activities for Seniors" (Geller, 2019).

4.3 Adapting Activities for Residents with Impairments

While activities are beneficial to all residents, some scheduled events may need to be modified to accommodate residents with physical or cognitive impairments. Exhibit 4.7 displays some suggestions to ensure residents with dementia are incorporated in activities. Despite any change in functional ability, residents with impairments get just as much—if not more, sometimes—out of activities and programming within a care center. This is especially true for residents with dementia who may be agitated and experiencing "behaviors" on a more routine basis, where redirection during an activity may provide a calming result.

Exhibit 4.7 Engaging Residents with Dementia or Cognitive Impairment through Activities in Care Centers
No matter if the resident is in a nursing home or assisted living center, it is important to engage those who may have a form of dementia or other cognitive impairment with activities that are regularly planned. Such involvement in facility programming can aid residents in preventing further cognitive decline and can ultimately improve quality of life. Goals for care centers to think about for inclusion of all residents include:

- Offer a number of activities each day that provide context with meaning tailored to individual residents, incorporating community-building, fun, and the ability to have choice in which activities the resident engages in.
- Activities should be designed to allow residents to actively participate, no matter their cognitive status (don't do the activity *for* the resident).
- Whatever the resident may prefer—including solitude, at times—should always be respected by staff members.

Adapted from the Alzheimer's Association Campaign for Quality Residential Care "Dementia Care Practice Recommendations for Assisted Living Residences and Nursing Homes" (2009).

Residents experiencing dementia often do best and participate more frequently in planned events when they are structured as smaller group activities (i.e., 4–9 people participating), where sound is kept at moderate levels so as to avoid overstimulation (Cohen-Mansfield et al., 2009). Additionally, staff members can successfully increase engagement of residents with more severe cognitive impairment when they model desired behavior from residents (Cohen-Mansfield et al., 2009). Activities which are tailored to a resident's particular interests and functional ability can also significantly improve behavioral outcomes for residents with dementia (Kolanowski et al., 2011). Although, for residents with dementia, "any type of activity improved outcomes over baseline" and tailored activities specifically "improved engagement, captured attention, and increased resident alertness" (Kolanowski et al., 2011).

Beyond the more traditional, planned, group activities that can be held within care centers, some facilities have created activity stations—sometimes called "life stations" or "life skills stations" (Warner Design Associates, 2017)—for residents with dementia who may wander about the building. These stations can be located throughout the building to increase resident engagement and provide activities to occupy care recipients' time. Such stations may include a desk with stationary, pens, envelopes, and other miscellaneous office items; a tool bench, with safe tools and non-harmful items to tinker with; a laundry area with an artificial-looking washing machine or dryer and clothes to fold in a basket; or a cradle or stroller with a doll that residents can hold or take care of, perhaps even with a rocking chair included. One large benefit to such stations is that they can often be created out of curated materials placed together in an existing corner or space within the care center, rather than requiring any structural modification of the building, allowing for customization and adaptation as new residents arrive that may be enticed by a different activity or "themed" station.

Another type of activity station that is beneficial for residents with cognitive impairments are Snoezelen rooms. Such rooms are created for residents to have multiple sensory experiences, featuring "pleasant surroundings, soothing sounds, captivating aromas, tactile experiences, massage, ... and gentle movement" (Snoezelen Multi-Sensory Environments, 2021). Care centers that have integrated Snoezelen into care for residents with dementia have improved resident well-being through enhanced moods, improved happiness, and greater enjoyment among residents who have used them. These rooms also increase adaptive behaviors, with residents engaging more with nurse aides and showing improved ability to formulate sentences and better convey their thoughts (Van Weert et al., 2005). In fact, Snoezelen rooms may have better effects on residents' mood and behavior than does reminiscence therapy (Baillon et al., 2004).

4.4 Religious and Spiritual Activities

As older adults near the end of their lives, many turn to their faith or spiritual beliefs—or return to what they may have once practiced or believed in—given concerns as to the afterlife or what happens to them upon death. This effect is more pronounced in retirement years and may wane, in some cases, as older adults become cognitively impaired and are unable to fully participate in religious services (Bengtson et al., 2015). For many residents, attendance at religious services or community engagement through faith-related events has been a staple of their life and is something they wish to continue engaging in upon admission to a care center, no matter their physical or cognitive impairment. Not only are religious beliefs important to many people (Brenan, 2018), but those who hold religious beliefs tend to experience higher levels of well-being (Villani et al., 2019). Many older adults receive comfort from their faith (Malone & Dadswell, 2018) in dealing with stressful life events, which can include transitioning to a care community from the home they lived in. While spirituality and religion has been argued as necessary to incorporate into the medical care given to older adults (Peteet et al., 2019), it is an essential component of quality of life for residents in care centers.

Some residents consider their spiritual health or faith as a "bedrock" of health, but a resident's spiritual or religious beliefs can have positive effects on their ability to cope with stressors, improve their mental health by combatting depressive or anxious feelings, and may lead to general feelings of optimism and purpose (Mackenzie et al., 2000). The effect of spirituality or religious beliefs on residents in rural care centers may be even more pronounced and underscores the importance of activities and programs in these areas that include more faith-based content for residents (Yoon & Lee, 2006). While many spiritual beliefs are predicated on thoughts of the self, a resident's religious beliefs and practices also provide comfort for many when experiencing loss of a loved one, especially a resident's spouse (Damianakis & Marziali, 2011).

Given that, it becomes even more important to ascertain a resident's religious beliefs and preferences upon admission and incorporate individualized spiritual and religious events into regularly scheduled activities in a care center. Residents often create or maintain a sense of community with others in their building through religious or spiritual activities, so many faith-based events in care communities are designed for groups to offer both spiritual nourishment as well as fellowship opportunities. Many contemporary facilities hold weekly religious services in their buildings, usually in a dedicated religious space, such as a chapel or synagogue (Fig. 4.6). While some care centers are affiliated with one faith or denomination (e.g., Catholic, Jewish), many try to deliver a variety of services to satisfy the diverse needs of all residents in their building. This can include inviting various clergy and spiritual leaders from the community into the building to use the chapel or other rooms for services, or to meet individually with residents in their rooms.

While many care centers have more formal religious services, some have incorporated religious and spiritual practices into traditional activities and programming, too. Some care centers plan bible studies or activities to discuss religious texts,

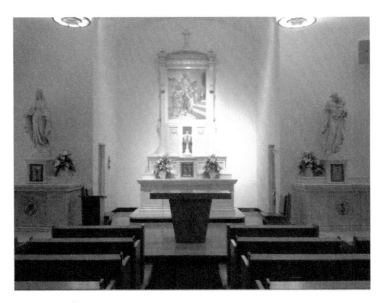

Fig. 4.6 The Chapel of Summa. Many care centers have constructed buildings with chapels and other spaces set aside for religious services, prayer groups, and bible study activities. Such chapels often are often "agnostic," in that the space can be used for multiple faiths or denominations to hold services for residents who practice and believe in a certain religion. During holidays, many care centers host religious or spiritual services or events and host family members of residents. This is particularly helpful for residents who are unable to safely leave the care center for various reasons. Photo Credit: PFAStudent at English Wikipedia

providing a quiet meeting space for residents who share similar spiritual or belief structures to gather and discuss their faith. Numerous care centers also host events near religious holidays, which are often times where family and friends of the resident may come to the care community to join the resident in the service or related activities. Facilities also incorporate religious services to honor the loss of a friend or fellow resident in the building. Having funeral services or memorials can greatly aid residents in the grieving process and provide a sense of closure, especially when family may be invited to share stories and reminisce during the event. Some care centers that have veterans as residents often do special services in conjunction with local VFW or American Legion chapters in the United States—titled "Military Funeral Honors Programs" in some states—to honor the deceased person and their military service (e.g., Wisconsin Department of Veterans Affairs, 2021).

With religious activities or celebrations, this also creates the potential to invite members of the community into the building, such as for "Secret Santa" events or with elementary school or middle school choirs performing for the residents. Additionally, it is important to note that some residents are unable to leave their room to attend services or activities. Some care centers have created a closed-circuit television channel to broadcast religious services or other activity programming directly into residents' rooms. In addition, it is becoming more common for community churches to use technology to broadcast their services on television, the radio, or even over social media channels. As care centers incorporate more technology and devices, this can create an opportunity for residents to virtually participate in the services of their home congregation, allowing them to maintain both their religious beliefs and practices and an external connection to a familiar community, which may bring them additional comfort and improve overall quality of life.

4.5   Essential Influencers

Supporting residents in their emotional and physical well-being, meaning, and purpose through ensuring they have ample opportunity to engage in stimulating and meaningful activities is an important responsibility for all staff, but some play an especially important role.

4.5.1   Activities Director

The staff member with the greatest ability to affect the quality, frequency, and variety of activities is the activities or therapeutic recreation director himself or herself. In some contemporary care communities, this role is titled a life enrichment coordinator or director, or a director of activities and wellness, given recent emphasis on complementary and alternative practices incorporated into activities and programming (e.g., deep breathing and mindfulness exercises). Generally speaking, this is the person responsible for planning and executing the programming within a facility, including arranging for guests to visit the care center, acquiring supplies for activities, coordinating external visits (if any), and overseeing other staff members in the facility that might assist with the events themselves. The activities director should work closely with the social workers or admissions staff to utilize detailed resident information and plan activities accordingly. Additionally, the director can better tailor activities by continually soliciting resident feedback on new activities, frequency, and even the scheduling during each day to enable more residents to attend (e.g., if activities are always scheduled during therapy sessions, it may preclude residents from attending that would enjoy the socialization and event).

4.5.2 Activity Aides and Volunteers

In larger care centers, there may be a person in charge of activities and wellness for residents, with numerous staff members deployed throughout the building that lead individual activities with residents. These staff members often aid in the design of activities that are tailored to specific resident preferences and desires, and they can also support greater specialization based on each person's unique talents, abilities, and interests. Aides can get to know the residents and directly solicit feedback on how to improve the activities offered. As aides know more about residents over time, they can also assist the director in planning events or tailoring existing events to accommodate any resident impairment (e.g., yoga activities may be modified to a chair yoga activity for some folks). Aides can also coordinate with therapy staff to thoughtfully incorporate any exercise programs within activities in a way that supports residents but also promotes resident enjoyment and participation.

Some care centers also seek out volunteers from the community to come in and assist with activities. This can include family members of the residents or other retired individuals that wish to give back or support a member from their neighborhood or faith community. Such volunteers can provide invaluable "person power" to staff activities and potentially bring in a new event to supply ample variety for programming each month. Volunteers can also help a care center feel more like "home" with familiar faces the residents remember from the community.

4.5.3 Social Workers

Other staff members that can aid in the planning of activities are those that are instrumental in collecting resident-specific data upon admission and during routine care conferences at the care center. Whoever assists with new admissions—potentially a social worker or admissions director role—can tailor welcome materials to include surveys or questionnaires about the resident, including a prior occupation, activities they enjoy, hobbies they may have had, and their spiritual beliefs and practices to tailor religious activities. This information can be included within care planning, where ongoing assessments can gauge residents' satisfaction with the offering of activities and inform new activities or modifications to existing events to more fully enable resident participation and engagement.

4.5.4 Therapists

Physical therapists (PTs) and occupational therapists (OTs) are also valuable staff members that influence the quality of activities. Especially for events that have physical components to them, PTs and OTs should be consulted to determine if any physical modifications are required to enhance resident participation and enjoyment (e.g., yoga that becomes chair yoga to aid with balance and fatigue from standing too long). Soliciting advice from OTs could also help individuals with cognitive impairment, such as those residents receiving rehabilitation following a stroke, to participate more fully. The incorporation of PTs and OTs in activities planning sessions can also ensure that activities align thoughtfully with residents' therapy plans, to enhance both the quality of care component as well as enhancing resident quality of life in the process.

4.5.5 Clergy

Lastly, with respect to religious and spiritual activities, the clergy or faith leaders for a given care community are essential influencers of this aspect of quality of life. As noted above, many older adults increase their spiritual or religious activities in later life, especially as the end of life approaches. Clergy and faith leaders may be directly employed by the care center or may be from the surrounding community and make visits to residents that were former parishioners. These faith leaders can help the activities director plan routine religious services in the building or establish bible study groups or smaller groups studying religious texts. They can also offer their services to individual residents, by bringing religious rituals (e.g., delivering weekly communion) directly to residents who have a harder time joining in group services, and can assist with individual counseling if a resident is in distress due to illness, emotional distress, or when near the end of life.

References

Altintas, E., De Benedetto, G., & Gallouj, K. (2017). Adaptation to nursing home: The role of leisure activities in light of motivation and relatedness. *Archives of Gerontology and Geriatrics, 70*, 8–13. https://doi.org/10.1016/j.archger.2016.12.004

Alzheimer's Association. (2009). *Dementia care practice recommendations for assisted living residences and nursing homes.* Campaign for Quality Residential Care. Retrieved from https://www.alz.org/media/documents/dementia-care-practice-recommend-assist-living- 1-2- b.pdf.

Baillon, S., Van Diepen, E., Prettyman, R., Redman, J., Rooke, N., & Campbell, R. (2004). A comparison of the effects of Snoezelen and reminiscence therapy on the agitated behaviour of patients with dementia. *International Journal of Geriatric Psychiatry, 19*(11), 1047–1052. https://doi.org/10.1002/gps.1208

Bellarmine University Veritas Society, School of Continuing and Professional Studies. (2021). *Veritas society.* Retrieved from https://www.bellarmine.edu/ce/veritas/

Bengtson, V. L., Silverstein, M., Putney, N. M., & Harris, S. C. (2015). Does religiousness increase with age? Age changes and generational differences over 35 years. *Journal for the Scientific Study of Religion, 54*(2), 363–379. https://doi.org/10.1111/jssr.12183

Björk, S., Lindkvist, M., Wimo, A., Juthberg, C., Bergland, Å., & Edvardsson, D. (2017). Residents' engagement in everyday activities and its association with thriving in nursing homes. *Journal of Advanced Nursing, 73*(8), 1884–1895. https://doi.org/10.1111/jan.13275

Brenan, M. (2018). *Religion considered important to 72% of Americans.* Retrieved from https://news.gallup.com/poll/245651/religion-considered-important-mericans.aspx

Cohen-Mansfield, J., Marx, M. S., & Werner, P. (1992). Observational data on time use and behavior problems in the nursing home. *Journal of Applied Gerontology, 11*(1), 111–121. https://doi.org/10.1177/073346489201100109

Cohen-Mansfield, J., Thein, K., Dakheel-Ali, M., & Marx, M. S. (2009). Engaging nursing home residents with dementia in activities: The effects of modeling, presentation order, time of day, and setting characteristics. *Aging and Mental Health, 14*(4), 471–480. https://doi.org/10.1080/13607860903586102

Crisis Prevention Institute, Dementia Care Specialists. (2015, August). *Life story questionnaire for more person-centered dementia care.* Retrieved from: https://www.crisisprevention.com/CPI/media/Media/Specialties/dcs/Life-Story- Questionnaire.pdf.

Daily Caring. (2021). *Chair Yoga for seniors: Reduce pain and improve health.* Retrieved from https://dailycaring.com/chair-yoga-for-seniors-reduce-pain-and-improve-health-video/

Damianakis, T., & Marziali, E. (2011). Older adults' response to the loss of a spouse: The function of spirituality in understanding the grieving process. *Aging and Mental Health, 16*(1), 57–66. https://doi.org/10.1080/13607863.2011.609531

Geller, H. (2019, October). *The benefits of intergenerational activities for seniors.* Elder Care Alliance. Retrieved from https://eldercarealliance.org/blog/benefits-intergenerational-programs/ .

Golden Carers. (2021). *Drum circle activity for the elderly.* Retrieved from https://www.goldencarers.com/drum-circle-activity-for-the-elderly/5032/

Harvard Health. (2019). *Exercise after age 70.* Retrieved from https://www.health.harvard.edu/staying-healthy/exercise_after_age_70

Honor Flight. (2021). *About us.* Retrieved from https://www.honorflight.org/about-us.html

Ibrahim, S. A. S., & Dahlan, A. (2015). Engagement in occupational activities and purpose in life amongst older people in the community and institutions. *Procedia – Social and Behavioral Sciences, 202*, 263–272.

It's Never Too Late (IN2L). (2021). *Our solution: Content.* Retrieved from https://in2l.com/our-solution/content/

Johs-Artisensi, J. L., Hansen, K. E., & Olson, D. M. (2020). Qualitative analyses of nursing home residents' quality of life from multiple stakeholders' perspectives. *Quality of Life Research, 29,* 1229–1238. https://doi.org/10.1007/s11136-019-02395-3

Kolanowski, A., Litaker, M., Buettner, L., Moeller, J., & Costa, P. T. (2011). A randomized clinical trial of theory-based activities for the behavioral symptoms of dementia nursing home residents. *Journal of the American Geriatrics Society, 59*(6), 1032–1041. https://doi.org/10.1111/j.1532-5415.2011.03449.x

Krause, N., Herzog, A. R., & Baker, E. (1992). Providing support to others and Well-being in later life. *Journal of Gerontology, 47*(5), P300–P311. https://doi.org/10.1093/geronj/47.5.P300

LeadingAge. (2021). *Resident engagement during social isolation.* Retrieved from https://leadingage.org/resident-engagement-during-social-isolation

Lumosity. (2021). *Brain games.* Retrieved from https://www.lumosity.com/en/brain-games/

Mackenzie, E. R., Rajagopal, D. E., Meilbohm, M., & Lavizzo-Mourey, R. (2000). Spiritual support and psychological Well-being: Older adults' perceptions of the religion and health connection. *Alternative Therapies in Health and Medicine, 6*(6), 37–45.

Malone, J., & Dadswell, A. (2018). The role of religion, spirituality and/or belief in positive ageing for older adults. *Geriatrics, 3*(2), 28. https://doi.org/10.3390/geriatrics3020028

Menec, V. H. (2003). The relation between everyday activities and successful aging: A 6-year longitudinal study. *Journals of Gerontology, Series B: Psychological Sciences and Social Sciences, 58*(2), S74–S82.

Music and Memory. (2012). *How to create a personalized playlist for your loved one at home.* Retrieved from https://alzheimer.ca/greybruce/sites/greybruce/files/documents/Music-and-Memory-How-to-create-a-personalized-playlist_Alzheimer-Society-Grey-Bruce.pdf

Music and Memory. (2021). *Music and the brain.* Retrieved from https://musicandmemory.org/resources/#power-of-music

MyElder. (2021). *Wii by Nintendo: An effective way for elders to exercise and have fun.* Retrieved from https://myelder.com/wii-by-nintendo-an-effective-way-for-elders-to-exercise-and-have-fun/

National Consumer Voice for Quality Long-Term Care. (2011). *Tips for building community involvement in long-term care facilities.* Retrieved from http://theconsumervoice.org/uploads/files/events/Tips-for-Building-Community-Involvement-.pdf

Peteet, J. R., Al Zaben, F., & Koenig, H. G. (2019). Integrating spirituality into the care of older adults. *International Psychogeriatrics, 31*(1), 31–38. https://doi.org/10.1017/S1041610218000716

Sit and Be Fit. (2021). *Seniors chair exercise programs.* Retrieved from https://www.sitandbefit.org/

Slettebø, Å., Sæteren, B., Caspari, S., Lohne, V., Rehnsfeldt, A. W., Heggestad, A. K. T., Lillestø, B., Høy, B., Råholm, M., Lindwall, L., Aasgaard, T., & Nåden, D. (2017). The significance of meaningful and enjoyable activities for nursing home resident's experiences of dignity. *Scandinavian Journal of Caring Sciences, 31*(4), 718–726. https://doi.org/10.1111/scs.12386

Snoezelen Multi-Sensory Environments. (2021). *Benefits and applications.* Retrieved from https://www.snoezelen.info/benefits-and-applications/

Substance Abuse and Mental Health Services Administration, United States Department of Health and Human Services. (2011). *A guide to promoting emotional health and preventing suicide in senior living communities.* Retrieved from: https://store.samhsa.gov/sites/default/files/d7/priv/guide.gettingstarted.pdf

Tellis-Nayak, V., Shiverick, B. N., & Hernandez, M. (2010). Where allies part ways and strangers converge: Nursing home performance in the eyes of residents, families, and state surveyors. *Seniors Housing and Care Journal, 18*(1), 3–19.

Thrive Center. (2021). *Social engagement.* Retrieved from https://www.thrivecenterky.org/social-engagement/

Van Weert, J. C. M., Van Dulmen, A. M., Spreeuwenberg, P. M. M., Ribbe, M. W., & Bensing, J. M. (2005). Behavioral and mood effects of Snoezelen integrated into 24-hour dementia care.

Journal of the American Geriatrics Society, 53(1), 24–33. https://doi.org/10.1111/j.1532-5415. 2005.53006.x

Villani, D., Sorgente, A., Iannello, P., & Antonietti, A. (2019). The role of spirituality and religiosity in subjective Well-being of individuals with different religious status. *Frontiers in Psychology, 10*, 1525. https://doi.org/10.3389/fpsyg.2019.01525

Warner Design Associates. (2017). *Utilizing life skills stations in memory care.* Retrieved from https://www.warnerdesignassociates.com/life-skills-stations-memory-care/

Wisconsin Department of Veterans Affairs. (2021). *Military funeral honors program.* Retrieved from https://dva.wi.gov/Pages/memorialsBurials/MilitaryFuneralHonors.aspx

Yoon, D. P., & Lee, E. K. O. (2006). The impact of religiousness, spirituality, and social support on psychological Well-being among older adults in rural areas. *Journal of Gerontological Social Work, 48*(3–4), 281–298. https://doi.org/10.1300/J083v48n03_01

Chapter 5
Environment and Surroundings

*Yes, your home is your castle, but it is also your identity and
your possibility to be open to others.* – David Soul

Abstract The physical environment influences quality of life for residents in long-term care, especially as it impedes or supports privacy and autonomy, and can particularly affect residents with dementia. The impact of the built environment and evidence-based design practices are explored, including physical design and re-design of rooms and communal spaces within facilities to promote a homelike environment. This can include the use of smaller spaces, as well as color and design strategies, to maximize resident independence and autonomy. Other content addresses residents' ability to personalize both their own living spaces and to have input into the communal spaces of their home. Additionally, strategic placement of seating options to facilitate socialization and physical activity are addressed, along with examining the value of outside spaces to support well-being and sensory engagement. Lastly, environmental recommendations to support residents with cognitive impairments are made, including environmental cuing, prevention of elopement, and activity stations to alleviate distress and promote engagement.

Keywords Homelike design · Medical model · Sense of home · Physical
environment · Memory impairment · Hospitality · Institutional · Resident bedrooms ·
Privacy · Personal belongings · Décor · Autonomy · Bathrooms · Communal spaces ·
Caregiver workspaces · Living spaces · Kitchen · Dining spaces · Shower · Tub
room · Spa · Comfortability · Lighting · Ambient noise · Safety · Outdoors ·
Wandering · Orientation · Wayfinding · Elopement

When care recipients are admitted to long-term care communities, it is expected their basic needs for shelter, nourishment, and health care will be met. When considering ways to enhance quality of life and well-being within care communities, a focus may be on changing operational practices, especially because administrators may have budgetary constraints that inhibit designs for new construction or remodeling. However, the physical environment plays an important role in resident quality of life, and care environments can be therapeutically designed or enhanced to facilitate improved health, safety, and well-being outcomes.

In recent decades, long-term care has shifted away from an institutional, medical model toward a more holistic model of care. Such culture change emphasizes dignity, independence, privacy, individualized care, stimulation, relationships, engagement, and well-being (Koren, 2010) that is provided in a more homelike environment. The physical environment of long-term living spaces includes the layout and functionality of space, as well as indoor and outdoor interior design and décor, which impacts several of these principles of care. Key factors from the "built environment" that most influence residents' sense of home include availability and composition of private and public spaces, personal belongings, technology, "look and feel", outdoor space, and geographic location (Eikelboom, 2017). Long-term care communities should be built on evidence-based strategies, designed to provide the best possible physical environment to support resident care and quality of life, while simultaneously encompassing design elements to support the efficiencies of caregiver staff.

5.1 Use of Homelike Design Principles

Long-term care communities are unique because they are both a person's home as well as a care facility, tasked with providing health and supportive care and often governed by significant regulation, much of which stems from a desire to protect vulnerable residents. Many care facilities were originally built mimicking the "medical model" design of hospitals which proliferated on the heels of post-World War II medical advances. Long-term care institutions were originally designed to focus on efficient processes in provision of care while minimizing staffing, equipment, and space needs to serve the maximum number of care recipients. This often meant buildings with multiple residents sharing rooms, kitchen and dining rooms structured with an assembly line mindset, and double-loaded corridors (e.g., hallways with resident rooms on each side, housing two to four residents each) with centralized nursing stations to maximize staff efficiencies and revenues.

Over time, lessons learned have demonstrated that meeting basic resident needs like food, shelter, and safety while prioritizing operational efficiencies over resident autonomy robs care recipients of their independence and well-being. Consumers have propelled the Culture Change movement by demanding more homelike environments for themselves and their loved ones. In some places, regulatory changes have also pushed to deinstitutionalize the structure, model, and physical environment of care communities to strengthen lifestyle autonomy (Verbeek, 2016), enhance well-being (Eikelboom, 2017), and decrease negative outcomes associated with traditional models of care (Wrublowsky, 2018).

A resident's sense of home develops gradually and is influenced by both psychological factors, including autonomy, and social factors, including relationships and activities (Rijnaard, 2016). Exhibit 5.1 highlights some factors that influence a resident's sense of home in a care center. A person's sense of home is more about a feeling than a place. Residents want the place they live to "feel like home" (Bowman, 2008), which refers to a feeling of comfortability, order, orientation, safety, and understanding. Home is where daily activities occur, conversations are had, stories and memories are created, bodies are nourished, interactions occur in living and dining areas, and outdoor spaces invigorate souls with nature and light. The architecture and design that influence the built environment also contribute to a resident's perception of their environment as homelike (Eikelboom, 2017).

Exhibit 5.1 Factors Influencing Sense of Home in Nursing Homes
Psychological Factors

- Sense of acknowledgement.
- Preservation of one's habits and values.
- Autonomy and control.
- Coping.

Social Factors

- Interaction and relationships with staff.
- Interaction with other residents.
- Interaction with family and friends.
- Interaction with pets.
- Activities.

The Built Environment

- The private space.
- The (quasi-) public space.
- Personal belongings.
- Technology.
- Look and feel.
- Outdoors and location.

Adapted from "The Factors Influencing the Sense of Home in Nursing Homes: A Systematic Review from the Perspective of Residents" (Rijnaard, 2016).

Domains such as meaningful relationships, autonomy, sense of community, the dining experience, and activities (Johs-Artisensi et al., 2020), among additional aspects such as comfort, safety, enjoyment, functionality, and spiritual well-being (Kane et al., 2003), are all quality of life factors that can either be enhanced or hampered by the physical environment (Cutler, 2008; Salonena et al., 2013). Although positive environments may not increase satisfaction when quality of care is good, negative environments may decrease satisfaction when quality of care is low (Andrade et al., 2016).

Many long-term care recipients experience some degree of memory impairment, either as part of a dementia process or, to a lesser degree, as a consequence of normal aging. This can impact their adjustment when transitioning from their original home to living in a care community. Beyond positively impacting quality of life, the built environments of care communities can be tailored to support therapeutic memory care and outcomes by reducing institutional elements which may exacerbate disruptive behavioral symptoms such as agitation, aggression, and restlessness (Wrublowsky, 2018).

5.1.1   Homelike and Hospitable Care

In some places, long-term care providers have slowly been replacing institutional models of care with newer models. One trend is to build "households" or "neighborhoods" within larger buildings to eliminate the double-loaded corridor that is a hallmark of the medical model. Some care centers have even constructed separate, self-contained homes as part of a larger campus, where each houses fewer than 25 residents. One such concept is referred to as the Green House model (The Green House Project, n.d.) (see Exhibit 5.2). The idea is these smaller houses have a residential look and feel, with their own kitchen, dining area, shared living spaces, and individual bedrooms but also incorporate a team of consistent staff who serve this smaller group of residents (Pioneer Network, 2011). The homes are furnished with residential furniture, bedrooms are decorated by residents and contain their personal items, and staff and residents prepare food and eat together in kitchen and dining areas, sitting around the table with food served family style in large bowls. Guests are welcome, and this homelike environment allows residents more autonomy, results in deeper relationships between peers and staff, and leads to an enhanced sense of home (Pioneer Network, 2011). Additionally, the administrator of one such model reports the cost of care in smaller homes with private rooms is equal to or less than the cost of care in traditional models (Bowman, 2008).

Exhibit 5.2 The Green House Project
32 states are home to 300 Green Houses, where 10–12 residents live in a housing center with a shared open kitchen, dining room, and a living room. Special cross-trained nursing assistants work exclusively in a single home, making meals, doing laundry, socializing, helping residents pursue their interests, and looking for early signs of health issues. The features that make these homes great places to live also have the benefit of offering better infection control mitigation strategies and have been found to reduce Medicare Part A hospitalizations by 30%.
Adapted from AARP's "10 Steps to Reform and Improve Nursing Homes" (Harrar et al., 2021).

Whether new builds or retrofits (i.e., remodeling floors or units into households within existing institutionally designed buildings), converting some areas to more residentially oriented shared spaces can include redecorating with homelike principles in mind. In so doing, the emphasis should be on looking as much like a home as possible, because it is easier for residents to feel less like a patient and more like they are in their own "home" if the environment reflects this (Shields, 2006). Attention should even be paid to exterior features. Although it may be easier to make a new small house look like just that from the outside, even a retrofitted household within an older building can be designed so that as one is approaching, features compatible with a home's exterior, such as porches, front doors, doorbells, porch lights, and mailboxes that then open up to interiors that also look and feel residential are visible. In these spaces, residents can find privacy in their own bedrooms or bathrooms, while gathering with peers, staff, or guests in common spaces to cook, eat, talk, laugh, and live.

Many long-term care communities serve not only long-term populations, for whom the space truly is home but increasingly, especially in skilled nursing facilities in the United States, also serve short-term populations who are there for only a few days, weeks, or months for rehabilitation or healing. These care recipients, while sharing many similar needs with longer-term residents, are not likely to want to supply their own furniture or spend significant time personalizing their space, with a goal of returning to their original home. Neither population prefers an institutional environment, so a functional and inviting environment best suits both. However, the short-term population may favor less of a homelike environment and rather something more akin to a hotel, with pleasant décor and furnishings provided, including guest seating, a desk or workspace, and other amenities to make their short stay comfortable while they heal and rehabilitate, continuing their normal routine as much as possible (Johs-Artisensi et al., 2021). A hotel-like approach, including elements such as a concierge-type resource book, toiletries, notepad and pens, clock, phone, television, wifi, and a place to store in-room snacks or beverages tend to be well-received by short-term clientele. Examples of hotel-like suites are provided in Exhibit 5.3.

Exhibit 5.3 Hotel-Like Suites are the New Nursing Home

"Luxury" is being used today to describe the environment of some skilled nursing facilities, making the experience resemble a hotel stay. The Health and Rehabilitation Center at Selfhelp in Chicago, Illinois offers plush robes, in-room dining, private suites, wifi and spa like services. The space was designed using calming colors, uplifting and encouraging artwork, lighting with a home-like sensibility, and cushioned flooring for added safety. The intent was to create a space that offered a strong sense of independence and dignity that can sometimes be lost after a decline in health. Their architects worked closely with the nursing and therapy teams, resulting in designs

(continued)

Exhibit 5.3 (continued)
focused on storage and convenience, while giving as much space as possible to residents.

Large private suites—with space for overnight guests, private bathrooms, and wheelchair accessible showers—are featured in each personal room. There are community rooms for dining, activities, and quiet spaces for residents to socialize and have private conversations with guests. Spacious therapy rooms, including a water therapy room for whirlpool treatments, lend a relaxing, spa-like look.

The hope is that environmental designs like updated therapy rooms, overnight accommodations for spouses, and barrier-free showers are features that will positively affect resident outcomes and quality of life.

Adapted from Selfhelp Home's "Hotel like suites are the new nursing home" (2016).

5.1.2   Resident Bedrooms

A key component of quality of life includes a quality living environment (Kane et al., 2004). This requires not just making space available but ensuring it feels homelike and residents can use it to engage in activities that will enhance their well-being. Through thoughtful, stealthy residential design strategies, necessary medical supplies or equipment can be concealed or disguised—for example, medications can be stored in bathroom cabinets and medical equipment behind wooden façades instead of storing it in plain view. If adequate square footage exists, rooms should be laid out with separate spaces for sleeping, leisure activities, and hosting guests. Residents should be able to visit with a friend or family member within their personal bedroom, with comfortable seating options that don't require the guest to sit on their bed. They should also be given adequate space and furniture for engaging in leisure activities, such as a television and a desk or fold-down table. They should have privacy for hosting guests, receiving medical or personal hygiene care, engaging intimacy or simply enjoying solitude, and should be able to be surrounded by their personal belongings.

5.1.2.1   Privacy

The desire for privacy emerges early in the life course (Wolfe, 1978) and persists throughout. Reasons demonstrating the importance of privacy are included in Exhibit 5.4. A sense of home for long-term care residents is augmented with access to private space. Autonomy is the likely driver for this desire, but relative to the built environment of long-term care, the strong desire for a private room is likely rooted in the opportunity to spend time alone, be surrounded by personal belongings, and create their own ambiance and experience, whether through personal decorations or how they choose to spend their time (Eikelboom, 2017). In addition, residents should have some control over not just what is in their space, but who is in it, and when; if anyone can barge in at any time, residents really don't have any privacy.

Exhibit 5.4 Reasons why Privacy Matters
- **Respect for Individuals**—Privacy is about respecting individuals. If someone violates your privacy it feels like they are saying, "I care about my interests, but I don't care about yours."
- **Reputation Management—How** we are judged by others affects our opportunities, relationships, and overall well-being. Privacy helps people protect themselves against troublesome judgments.
- **Maintaining Appropriate Social Boundaries**—We need places of solitude to retreat to, where we are free of the gaze of others in order to relax and feel at ease.
- **Trust**—In relationships we depend upon trusting the other party. When trust is breached in one relationship, it may make us more reluctant to trust in other relationships.
- **Control Over One's Life**—One of the hallmarks of freedom is having autonomy and control over our lives, and we can't have that if important decisions about us are being made in secret without our awareness or participation.
- **Freedom of Thought, Speech, and Activity**—Privacy is key to freedom of thought and protecting our ability to hold and speak even unpopular messages. It protects our ability to associate with other people and engage in activities of our choosing.
- **Ability to Change and Have Second Chances**—People are not static; they change and grow throughout their lives. Privacy nurtures our ability to have a second chance, reinvent oneself, grow and improve.
- **Not Having to Explain or Justify Oneself**—We may do things which, if judged from afar by others lacking complete knowledge or understanding, may seem odd or embarrassing or worse. It is a heavy burden to constantly wonder what we do will be perceived by others.

Adapted from Teach Privacy's "10 Reasons Why Privacy Matters" (Solove, 2014).

Living with strangers during adulthood is less common, so the possibility of being assigned a roommate when moving into a long-term care community can be a source of anxiety for many. Care recipients may worry about their ability to have privacy and also whether they will have adequate space, get along with a new person, have conflicts managing lifestyle choices, or how to avoid disturbing a roommate.

Private rooms (or at least having fewer roommates) are associated with better quality of life, in part because the more people who share a room, the less space there is for privacy and activity (Kane et al., 2004) and the more their personal environment will be disrupted by environmental noise and light, visitors, or caregivers. Rooms with multiple residents are often referred to, oxymoronically, as "semi-private," but are more aptly named "shared-rooms." Although private rooms may not suit everyone, as some might experience increased isolation or reduced emotional support (Salonena et al., 2013), they are strongly preferred by most care recipients. Private rooms have been shown to enhance operational efficiencies, improving both health and psychosocial well-being outcomes (Calkins & Cassella, 2007), including reducing stress (Salonena et al., 2013).

A typical long-term care resident room, whether private or shared, contains space for resting and sleeping, personal and social space, and a toileting area. The ideal space is a private room with an attached bathroom, preferably with large, low windows and wide doors, making it easy to move in one's own furniture and set items on windowsills, enjoy ample natural light, and have no roommate to disturb. It could be constructed with built-in shelving to display personal items or unique alcoves that offer the illusion of separate sleeping and social spaces within a single room.

In shared rooms, ideally there will be some delineation to designate which sleeping space belongs to each resident. It is common to see ceiling-mounted privacy curtains in shared rooms, which can be pulled when a roommate desires privacy. However, while a cloth curtain temporarily obstructs one's line of vision, it does not block sounds of televisions, conversations of guests or caregivers, or the use of a bedside commode. A privacy curtain is better than nothing at all, but it certainly isn't sufficient to preserve dignity and maximize quality of life. If shared rooms are to exist, creative designs can enhance the level of privacy. Shared spaces can be designed slightly larger, with partial or half walls or dual-sided bookcases between the two sides of the room to give more privacy while still sharing a common bathroom or sitting and workspace areas. Such bookcase-style partitions can also be used to display personal belongings of each resident in their respective sleeping space. Even the design of privacy-enhanced shared spaces can be thoughtful, with ideal designs not only affording each resident private space, but structuring them such that residents, caregivers, and guests can enter each residents' space without trespassing through the other's area.

5.1.2.2   Personal Belongings

Beyond private room preferences, care recipients have also been demanding more space and storage (Brawley, 1997). Bedrooms can provide privacy and a personal domain that strengthens self-identity when residents are allowed to personalize their own spaces with décor, furnishings, clothing, and possessions. These contribute to residents' sense of calm and research shows they can reduce stress and anxiety (Wrublowsky, 2018). Care recipients' well-being is enhanced when their space contains preferred items such as a comfortable chair, television or computing devices, horizontal workspace (e.g., to use for hobbies, puzzles, crafts, writing), or a small refrigerator. These accoutrements allow residents to use their personal space to engage in hobbies, visiting, and other leisure activities, promoting a more homelike feel (Kane et al., 2004).

Exhibit 5.5 Why "Stuff" Matters

Our relationship with "stuff" starts early. By age two, we begin to understand that we can own something, possess it as if a part of ourselves. As our lives unfold, our things embody our sense of selfhood and identity still further, becoming external receptacles for our memories, relationships, and travels. Beyond shoring up our sense of identity, our possessions allow us to signal something about ourselves to other people. As our belongings accumulate, becoming more infused with our identities, so their preciousness increases.

As with human relationships, the attachments to our things deepen with the passage of time. Older adults are often surrounded by possessions that have followed them through good times and bad, across continents and back. These possessions can be a particular comfort for older people who have to leave their homes and enter residential care, because cherished possessions often provided a vital link to memories, relationships, and former selves, helping foster a sense of continuity. After a person dies, many of their most meaningful possessions become family heirlooms, seen by those left behind as forever containing the lost person's essence.

Adapted from The Psychologist's "The Psychology of Stuff and Things" (Jarrett, 2013).

Having personal belongings is essential for developing and maintaining a sense of home (Eikelboom, 2017). There is an empowering element of autonomy in "nesting"—personalizing one's environment with familiarity to support self-identity (Falk et al., 2013)—and having a say in what one's environment will look like. Exhibit 5.5 discusses the importance of "stuff" for older adult residents. When beloved items from the resident's life are present in their environment, sentimental memories are evoked, helping them feel at home. If residents are surrounded by pictures of their loved ones, it helps them feel connected to family and friends. When communities allow residents to personalize their own spaces by bringing furniture, bedspreads, curtains, lamps, photos, or other items of emotional value (Fig. 5.1), they take on a role in creating their own home, creating a positive emotional attachment to their environmental surroundings that enhances their comfortability.

People are used to choosing their home décor so, when possible, residents should be allowed to choose paint colors, have a say in how furniture and belongings are arranged, and dictate the decoration of the interior of their room. Families play a large role in assisting residents with personalization of their rooms. They may be involved in selecting and moving furniture and personal belongings and can help the resident to decorate and get settled in their new space upon admission. For exterior design considerations, when someone approaches a resident's room, this is the first

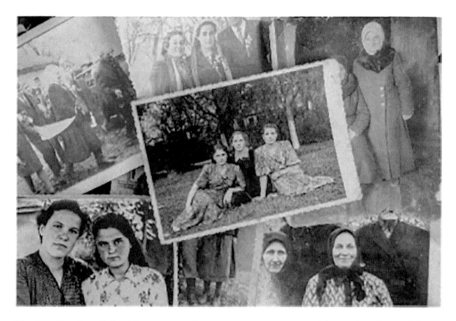

Fig. 5.1 Family relationships are very important to many care recipients. A collage of family photos, displayed in their room, can help a resident feel connected to family and friends. Photo Credit: Evgeniya Visochina

impression they have of the resident's space and, by extension, them. Residents may wish to decorate their exterior door to indicate their hospitality, celebrate seasonal holidays, or show off their own artwork or crafts. Some care communities have made room exteriors feel even more homelike by coupling room numbers with conventional street naming for various households or hallways, such as 406 Pinecone Lane or 502 Honeysuckle Hollow. Personalization of room exteriors also assists cognitively declined residents with wayfinding, as shown in Exhibit 5.6.

Exhibit 5.6 Personalized Doors Assist with Wayfinding
Residents at Nashwaak Villa in Stanley, New Brunswick, Canada, can personalize their doors with non-flammable, washable large vinyl decals from the Holland company True Doors. The decals engage residents and remind them of their past while also helping them navigate the care facility, which can often look alike and lead to confusion for residents who have trouble with wayfinding. It empowers residents with choice and stimulates memories of doors from residents' pasts.

Residents, sometimes with the help of their family, can choose a door decal from among 400 options or provide a photo of a door that was important to them. One resident has a decal of the door of the church where her daughter

(continued)

> **Exhibit 5.6** (continued)
> was married. For many residents, their personalized door gives them both a sense of home and security.
>   *Adapted from iAdvance Senior Care's "Personalized Doors Help Residents with Dementia to Find Their Way" (Stempak, 2017).*

5.1.2.3 Autonomy Over Personal Environment

Beyond what their personal space looks like, residents should also have some autonomy to control the ambient aspects of their environment, such as adjusting the temperature of their room, using an air freshener of their choice, listening to music, or having a television on. This can be especially challenging in a shared room situation, but manually closing vents or running a fan, or using wireless headphones, are options that can mitigate environmental roommate conflicts while supporting individual autonomy. Technology can also be useful in creating a homelike environment and enhancing autonomy. Residents gain access to the outside world and information with an internet-equipped computing device and independence with "smart" technology-equipped rooms to "ask Alexa" to open their shades, turn on the television, read them the morning news, or call their daughter.

5.1.2.4 Bathrooms

Residents prefer not to share bathrooms for the same reasons they favor private rooms. People engage in intimate, personal, private activities in their bathrooms and older adults may find the process of receiving assistance with toileting and bathing to be both physically and emotionally taxing. As individuals age, they may need faster access to a toilet. Incontinence affects nearly three-quarters of long-term care residents and has significant psychological and social impacts, majorly limiting quality of life. Incontinence episodes, and associated anxiety about them, can be reduced when toilets are visibly and easily accessible to residents and spaces have been designed with appropriate ergonomics, adequate space for wheelchairs and transfers, and ample grab bars (Wrublowsky, 2018).

   Ideally, a resident's primary sleeping and living space should be in close proximity to a toilet, as well as relative proximity to bathing facilities. Occasionally, when distance to a toilet is too far, a commode is placed in the living or sleeping space for convenience. Careful consideration should be given to such a decision, especially in a shared room, because while this may be beneficial in meeting a resident's physical need for elimination and reducing incontinence anxieties, it risks being a dignity issue by medicalizing the environmental living space.

   Personal bathrooms with showers (Fig. 5.2) eliminate the potential dignity issue of transporting residents (sometimes undressed, just covered by a sheet) through public spaces, enhance infection control by limiting exposure to other residents'

Fig. 5.2 At the Michael
J. Fitzmaurice State
Veterans Home, adjacent
resident bathrooms use an
open-concept, European
design, offering plenty of
space for maneuvering
equipment and multiple
caregivers, as well as an
accessible shower. An
attached bathroom off one's
personal room offers
convenience, reduces
incontinence concerns, and
offers privacy and dignity to
the bathing process. Photo
Credit: U.S. Department of
Veterans Affairs

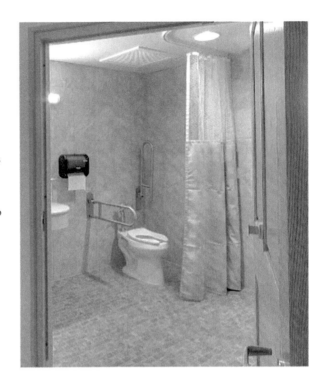

waste, and allow for easier cleansing in the event of incontinence soiling
(Wrublowsky, 2018). Although maintaining dignity and privacy is challenging
when one needs caregiver assistance with bathing, it should always be done without
a roommate present or another resident simultaneously being bathed in the same
space.

In an ideal situation, each resident is afforded a private bathroom with toileting
and showering facilities. For accessibility, a European design which utilizes the
entire washroom as a showering area can be employed. Some buildings may offer
private bathrooms with showers, supplemented by communal spas where more
comfortable bathing services may be provided. Even if showering facilities cannot
be provided in private bathrooms, having access to a private latrine and sink for
toileting and hygiene is highly desirable. Occasionally, buildings are designed with
private or shared rooms having a connecting bathroom shared among multiple
residents. Although this is preferable to a communal bathroom down the hall,
many residents still express a preference for their own private bathroom.

5.1.3 Design of Communal Spaces

A well-designed physical environment for long-term care recipients can balance the need to support socialization, mobility, activity, and autonomy while also ensuring safety. As noted previously, peer relationships are important for quality of life, so it is essential that residents are encouraged to spend time out of their personal rooms to engage with others (Fig. 5.3). To enable this, it is important that public spaces be designed with clear signaling about usage expectations. If an environment is too sterile, even if nicely appointed, it may suggest the space is for show rather than for use. Strategies such as personalizing living spaces with carpeting rather than tile and displaying photographs of the people who live there lend an ambiance of it being a true "living room" rather than simply a public lobby. Generally, smaller spaces with lower resident-density tend to feel more homelike than larger, less personal spaces (Eikelboom, 2017). Especially for those who live in shared rooms, engaging in preferred leisure activities, making phone or video calls, watching television, and hosting guests are functions that may also need to occur outside their bedrooms, so it is essential that adequate communal spaces accommodate a broad array of residents' psychosocial needs.

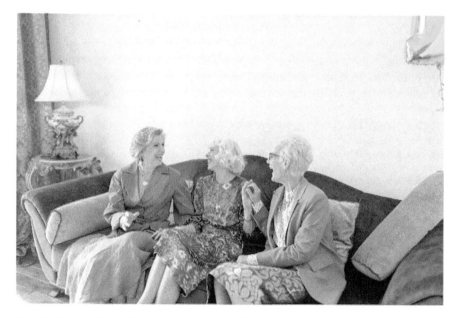

Fig. 5.3 Relationships with peers are instrumental in creating a sense of community. Assisted living residents gather in a public sitting room to enjoy each other's fellowship and conversation. Photo Credit: Yaroslav Shuraev

5.1.3.1   Caregiver Workspace

Besides meeting residents' environmental needs, it is important to think about how and where the staff spend their time. Ideally, resident rooms are physically designed to minimize the intrusion of caregivers in residents' personal space. For example, the use of dual-sided laundry cupboards allows caregivers to retrieve dirty laundry or linens from hallways, while residents, family, and personal caregivers can access them from the resident's personal bedroom or bathroom. Although caregivers spend significant time in residents' rooms, they also need workspace when not providing direct care and assistance to residents. A recent trend has been removing institutional-looking nursing stations from the center of care floors, but this must be balanced with creating too many private spaces where staff are tucked away from residents so that staff are visible and easily approachable (Eikelboom, 2017). Practicality or various regulations may dictate the presence of "nursing stations," but thoughtful design options can help avoid the too common scenario of staff hidden behind the counter with residents "parked" in front, unable to see above the counter from wheelchair level. If centrally located nursing stations remain present, they should be designed low and open, surrounded by seating options and wheelchair space to allow for residents to congregate with accessibility to staff without obstructing walkways (Fig. 5.4). If a large central station is not required, an alternative is multiple smaller desks scattered throughout the building with workspace for computers and paperwork, coupled with cabinet storage. These smaller workstations can have adjacent, comfortable seating for a few residents. In traditionally designed buildings with long corridors, smaller workstations can be placed midway down each corridor or, in household-style models, they can be tucked into dining or living room spaces (Cutler, 2008). Removing the visual barrier of a counter between residents and staff promotes resident-staff relationships, which are critical to resident well-being. These design considerations contribute to an environment that retains the homelike feel for residents, while also adapting to

Fig. 5.4 At the Michael J. Fitzmaurice State Veterans Home, the nursing station was designed with low counters that residents' can see over, even from a wheelchair, with ample comfortable seating in the adjacent public space. Photo Credit: U.S. Department of Veterans Affairs

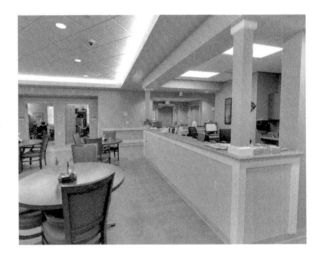

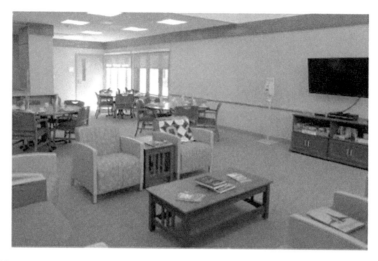

Fig. 5.5 At Veterans Homes of California in Fresno, seating is set up in conversational pods, with available books, games, and puzzles, to encourage socialization and activity in common areas. Photo Credit: U.S. Department of Veterans Affairs

staff's need to perform caregiving responsibilities unobtrusively but efficiently in the residents' home.

5.1.3.2   Living, Lounging, and Activity Spaces

Communal spaces where residents can congregate, socialize, and engage in activities are essential. Ideally, there will be multiple, unique spaces available within the care community for such purposes. Comfortable and functional furniture, with an eye toward safety, socialization, and leisure activities, should be included (Fig. 5.5). Furniture with a residential look, comfortable seats that still promote residents self-transferring, and padded armrests will encourage their use. Having a variety of seating options suitable for people of diverse heights and builds will assure comfort for all body types. To facilitate relationships, arranging seating into smaller group-ings or pods can encourage one on one or small group conversations with peers, visitors, or staff.

> **Exhibit 5.7 Tips for Integrating Cats into Nursing Homes**
> **Allow Adjustment Time**—Because cats may be skittish when transitioning to a new home, try to keep their surroundings calm during the adjustment period. Limit their territory initially and let them get used to the facility slowly.
> **Provide a Safe Home Base**—Set cats up with a home base, where litter boxes and food and water dishes can be made available, in a common area near a

(continued)

Exhibit 5.7 (continued)
cat-loving resident's room, if possible. Cats may be slightly cautious at first, but attention from residents is likely to ease their transition. Eventually cats should be content and happy to hang out in the common area, patrol the hallway, and visit residents in their rooms.

Choose Cats Suited to This Important Work—Adult cats may be best suited, so their dispositions can be known—look for cats who are calm, gentle, and enjoy being held and petted. The connection between a facility pet and the residents can bring diversion, interest, and happiness to residents' days.

Clearly Assign Responsibilities—Make sure it is understood who is providing care for the cats (e.g., feeding, cleaning litterboxes, veterinary care, shots, claw trimming). Often times activities staff provide the main care, although other staff and residents may also assume cat caregiver roles.

Ensure Safety of Cats and Residents—While you must ensure that cats don't harm residents (by choosing cats with good dispositions), you also want to make sure that residents don't harm cats, so keep cats away from potentially aggressive residents, or those who are unaware of their actions or their trength.

Adapted from Fear Free Pets' "How Cats Enhance a Nursing Home Setting" (Holm, n.d.).

Beyond the space itself, stocking the room with life-enriching features also benefits residents (Cutler, 2008). This may include telephones (especially important for those without a personal phone line in their bedroom), televisions, large-print reading materials, daily newspapers, or a community pet (Fig. 5.6). Exhibit 5.7 offers practical suggestions to incorporate a cat into a nursing home or care center environment. Due to space constraints, many care communities have what is termed a "multi-purpose room." While a better option than no communal space, it may be less inviting when the same room and furnishings are used for dining, activities, church services, and other events, especially because different social activities likely call for different furniture. For example, dining or playing cards often occurs around

Fig. 5.6 Pets can bring comfort, affection, friendship, activity, and a sense of purpose to residents in care centers. Here a residential care recipient pets a beloved care community pet. Photo Credit: Matthias Zomer

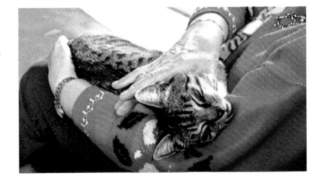

a table with more rigid chairs but socializing or watching television is more relaxing when seated in comfortable furniture, such as an overstuffed chair or couch. When a room must serve multiple purposes, interior design furnishings can increase ambiance and functionality. For example, dining tables can be hydraulicly raised to the ceiling or folded away and stored behind a façade when not in use if the room serves alternative purposes between meals. Even if tables cannot be removed, a varied ambiance can be created for different activities. For example, a mix of comfortable seating and tables supporting socializing, games, and movie watching during the day are appropriate and, at mealtimes, tables could be adorned with tablecloths or centerpieces to signal transformation from use as a lounge back to the dining room. Whether multi-purpose or a designated lounge, segmenting a room into delineated spaces for conversation, television watching, puzzles, or other activities allows these intentional spaces to feel more purposeful and inviting.

Additional design elements to support residents' quality of life include access to amenities that offer enrichment and fellowship opportunities beyond their bedrooms. These spaces may include chapels or meditation spaces, libraries or mobile book carts, gift or sundry shops, bistro cafe or coffee shop-type entities for snacks and socializing, beauty shops, movie theaters, fitness centers, or even daycare facilities for staff members that might offer the opportunity for intergenerational programming (see Exhibit 5.8 for examples of incorporating a preschool or daycare within a care center for older adults). Where regulations permit, even a residential-style laundry room could be considered, which could have folding tables and seating so that a resident could have a family member assist them in washing their own clothes. These kinds of spaces support purposeful activity for residents, giving them meaning, socialization opportunities, and a sense of contribution or purpose. Care communities may also expand their physical space to offer needed health care services for residents, such as dental care, dialysis, or infusion centers. Some facilities have adopted a "town square" model, many of these amenities to meet social gathering needs of care recipients, and offering accessible restrooms, escort services, and general staff supervision to encourage their use (Cutler, 2008) (Fig. 5.7).

Exhibit 5.8 Benefits of a Long-Term Care-Based Preschool or Daycare
When seniors enter long-term care communities it can leave them feeling isolated and cause them to miss out on some of the benefits that accompany being around younger people. Care facilities often have staffing challenges, and with caregivers often being women—many times young women with children—establishing a care community-based preschool or daycare can offer a multitude of benefits:

- **An onsite daycare is a useful staff recruitment and retention tool—the convenience of having your child's daycare at the same place you work can not be beat, especially if staff are offered a discount.**

(continued)

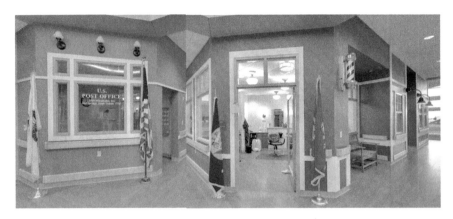

Fig. 5.7 At the Michael J. Fitzmaurice State Veterans Home, the "town square" contains unique features such as a post office and a beauty shop, giving the facility more of a local community feel. This type of design brings elements of exterior architecture indoors, to give the feeling of being on a street. Photo Credits: U.S. Department of Veterans Affairs

Exhibit 5.8 (continued)
- **Kids learn to be comfortable around people of other generations—** spending time with seniors as youngsters allows children to develop open minds about older adults and they will grow up treating seniors respectfully and with compassion.
- **Spending time with kids helps seniors fight off loneliness—**Spending time with kids is a clear antidote to loneliness. Kids bring excitement, creativity, and interesting ideas and give seniors an opportunity for fun, connection, and laughter.
- **Having kids around makes seniors more active—**Staying active and engaging in social opportunities is a key to living longer and enjoying life. Kids move, play, and exude energy and can be a conduit to getting seniors chatting, playing, and enjoying themselves.
- **Kids don't care about the signs of dementia—**Kids have more patience than adults. They don't mind repeating themselves or notice frustrating changes in behavior. Because they are still learning what "normal" is, a person with signs of dementia is just another person to them.

Adapted from Senior Advisor's "5 Benefits of Putting a Preschool in a Nursing Home" (Hicks, n.d.).

Finally, practical design considerations should also be integrated, for example, ensuring resident access to nearby toilets. Avoiding incontinence is of great consequence to most residents, and a lack of easy toilet access (nearby, unlocked, and accessible) in common spaces is a common resident complaint (Cutler, 2008) and a deterrent to them leaving their rooms to socialize. Likewise, throughout the building, residents need space to walk around or use assistive mobility devices as a leisure activity in and of itself. This requires safety devices such as handrails, hallways free of clutter, well-maintained flooring surfaces, ambulation surfaces that promote mobility, and a design that allows them someplace to move continuously. It is preferred that indoor walking spaces for resident exercise and mobility are designed either with a destination or as a loop, rather than a series of dead ends (Eikelboom, 2017).

5.1.3.3   Kitchen and Dining

In a "small home" or household model, one significant advantage is the presence of a homelike kitchen and dining space for use by a smaller group of residents. Smaller dining rooms with family-style dining rather than institutional line service enhance the perception of belonging (Eikelboom, 2017). Individuals may have a regular spot at the table or a preferred plate or glass which helps the communal dining experience feel more personal. For kitchens located within the household, breakfasts or snacks can be made to order or stored on the unit. Hot food for other meals, as well as food supplies to stock the kitchen, can be brought up from the main facility kitchen. With availability of a homelike kitchen, this can lead to residents eating regular meals at their leisure and enjoying coffee and conversation around the table much like they would have in their own homes.

Even facilities located in older medical-model buildings can be renovated with more modern design principles. For example, a long, double-loaded corridor wing could be converted by remodeling the first resident rooms on each side of the hallway into a lounge, nursing workstation, or dining room and kitchen, to create a household-type model on each wing (Cutler, 2008). Even in more traditionally designed facilities, offering smaller dining locations spread throughout libraries, sitting rooms, sunrooms, or lounges can foster autonomy, with residents perhaps opting for breakfast in one location and lunch in another, or sharing different meals with different peer groups. Another option, besides traditional dining rooms or household kitchens, is to have a bistro or café available to residents outside of mealtimes, where snacks are available on demand. Decentralizing large dining rooms is also beneficial for accommodating residents with mobility challenges, as it is often challenging for staff to transport all residents to a central location for meals simultaneously. This leads to residents spending extra time waiting for transport, being transported, and arriving early to the dining room with more waiting commencing, adding boredom and monotony to their lives, and detracting from their quality of life.

It should not be underestimated how important mealtimes are to residents, so facilities should do all they can to enhance the décor of the physical environment. Environmental features that create a pleasant ambiance and enhance the dining experience include amenities such as windows in the dining room, pictures or artwork on the walls, the use of tablecloths or placemats, centerpieces, and menus in readable print sizes. One facility, intent on providing a special dining experience, built the dining room with high ceilings, adorned it with beautiful draperies and furniture, and had unlocked, nicely appointed bathrooms adjacent to the room. Waitstaff in crisp uniforms serve the meal at tables with linens and centerpieces, using porcelain plates, stainless flatware, and stemmed water goblets for a restaurant-like dining experience.

Finally, regardless of the kitchen and dining meal arrangements, there should be access to a homelike kitchen for resident use, whether for leisure activities or hosting guests. The ability to engage in an activity that one may have participated in daily for their whole lives is rewarding and reminiscent of home, for many. This also offers additional benefits to other care recipients, such as the smell of fresh baked cookies making the environment feel more homelike and may even stimulate other residents' appetites. This could even pique other residents' interest in coming out to the communal area to see what is going on or join in on the activity, leading to engagement and relationship building. Exhibit 5.9 presents the benefits from activities focusing on food for residents with dementia.

Exhibit 5.9 Benefits of Food-Based Activities for People with Dementia
The sight of fruit attractively presented on a platter, the smell of freshly brewed coffee, the crunch of toast: these are all examples of how food can stimulate our senses. For people with dementia—especially those who may be losing interest in food and participating in mealtimes—activities that focuses on stimulating the senses could be the key to encouraging them to eat or being able to enjoy food again. The smell of food, such as freshly baked bread, is a powerful way of stimulating appetites and conversation. For some, an activity that encourages sharing of memories related to food may be a powerful and positive experience. For others, it may be that simply being given the job of laying the table makes them feel more involved with—and positive about—the mealtime experience.
   Adapted from the Social Care Institute for Excellence's "Activities for People with Dementia Based Around Food".

5.1.3.4   Shower and Tub Rooms or "Spas"

Bathing is a necessary activity for care recipients, but rather than it being a relaxing experience, for many it threatens their dignity and serves as a source of agitation for both residents and staff (Barrick et al., 2008). Ideally, residents have a bathroom containing both a toilet and a shower within the privacy of their own room. If having an accessible bathtub is not practical in private bathrooms, having a nicely appointed communal tub room or mobile tub system, available to facilitate choice, is essential. However, when communal showers or bathing rooms are necessary, they should be designed thoughtfully and with resident dignity at the forefront of consideration. These rooms should be conveniently located but also placed such that frequently, publicly used corridors are avoided. Some care communities have started by renaming their bathing rooms as "spas," whose new name dictates a different orientation to design and ambiance. An example of a low-cost "spa" renovation is described in Exhibit 5.10. Too often bathing spaces are located on interior halls, lacking natural light, and feeling dark and dank, often compounded by practices that allow the communal bathing room to double as storage. These rooms should have decorative lighting fixtures, and appropriate décor, color, and accouterments. It may be beneficial to have a toilet and sink located within bathing spaces in case toileting is necessary during the bathing process. Beyond a large shower or whirlpool tub option, an ideal spa room might also include a shampoo bowl, mirrors, and comfortable seating, where staff or family members could assist an individual in shampooing and styling their hair, without the need for a full shower (Cutler, 2008). Amenities, such as heat lamps, heated floors, and towel warmers, can add warmth and comfort with a sense of luxuriousness. Provision of aromatherapy scents can help to create a calmer, more spa-like experience, especially if residents can choose their preferred scent, which can help residents look forward to the experience (see Exhibit 5.11). Mirrors in spa rooms should be built on a slight tilt so residents' reflections can be seen from a seated or wheelchair position to help residents self-perform their own hygienic practices, where possible, as it is difficult to maintain a sense of identity without seeing one's own reflection.

Exhibit 5.10 A "Spa" at the Monastery

What was once a sparse, dark hallway of a nuns' monastery, labeled "the infirmary" underwent a major facelift as part of a culture change reorientation. One such room that benefitted from the renovation was once called the "tub room" but it was rebranded as "the spa" prior to their grand reopening. The makeover was completed on a tight budget, with shelving and décor largely repurposed and repainted from garage sale finds, although a grant was received to purchase a new whirlpool tub, a towel warmer, and a small oil diffuser. The old tub room (which seemingly doubled as a storage room) was cleaned out, and the whirlpool tub was installed. Paints in light blues and greens and decorations with a beach theme adorned the walls. One tall, narrow shelving unit held a series of shoeboxes covered in contact paper, each labeled and filled with individual residents' preferred soaps and shampoos. Screw hooks were mounted to the wall to hold residents' robes, clothing, and damp towels. A wheelchair accessible countertop with a tilted mirror was included, so residents could see their reflections, while seated, as their caregiver brushed their hair after a bath. A towel warming rack was mounted on one wall, lending warmth to the space. An essential oil diffuser sat on a shelf, and residents were encouraged to select their favorite scent at the start of bath time. The moods of the residents were palpably more cheerful following the makeover of their living and bathing space.

Exhibit 5.11 Aromatherapy Makes "Scents"

Although essential oils and aromatherapy should never replace medical treatment in a care facility, studies are beginning to show they may have some positive benefits as a complimentary therapy to reduce stress and improve mood among residents and staff. Their use can be incorporated in a variety of ways: beyond diffusing into the air, they can be used during hand massages, while bathing, in compresses, as part of a hair and skin care regimen, or as steam inhalations. Some common oils and their primary effects include:

Essential oil class	Primary effect	Example oils
Mints	Energizing	Spearmint, wintergreen
Citrus	Uplifting	Tangerine, lemon
Spices	Warming, grounding, soothing	Myrrh, clary sage, clove
Herbs and grasses	Warming, energizing, renewing	Spikenard, thyme, rosemary
Trees	Grounding, soothing	Eucalyptus, cedarwood, cypress
Florals	Calming	Lavender, geranium, ylang ylang

Oils and effects adapted from American Nurse's "Using Aromatherapy in the Clinical Setting: Making Sense of Scents" (Reynolds, et al., 2018)

5.1.4   Environmental Comfortability

To feel like a home, a care center needs to look like a home and be comfortable in its architecture, interior design, and upkeep. To feel comfortable, the environment should be tidy and odor-free, but residents do not want their long-term care environment to look and feel like a hospital (Eikelboom, 2017). Beyond addressing resident preferences for adequate space, physical comfort of residential furnishings, and a homelike environment, a comfortable environment will also engage the senses with pleasant sights and colors, thoughtful exposure to light, and some autonomy over ambient noise and temperature.

The use of color and contrast can impact seniors' functionality, safety, and mood. Exhibit 5.12 shows the effects of various colors of wall paints on residents in care centers. Using complementary color palettes to select color combinations that are pleasing to the eye or selecting certain colors to engender a certain tone or mood (Yildirim et al., 2007) creates a pleasant space that promotes well-being. In addition, the thoughtful selection of contrasting hues can also play a role in accommodating vision changes or memory care issues (Bowman, 2008).

Exhibit 5.12 How Room Color Affects Mood

Color	Moods it can convey:
Red	• Raise energy. • Intense. • Shown to raise blood pressure, speed, respiration, and heart rate.
Orange	• Evokes excitement and enthusiasm. • Promotes activity.
Yellow	• Reminds of joy of sunshine. • Communicates happiness.
Pink	• Associated with love and kindness. • Boosts creativity.
Green	• Has a calming effect. • Relieves stress.
Blue	• Soothing. • Lowers blood pressure. • Slows respiration and heart rate.
Purple	• Elegance and sophistication for darker purples. • Relaxation for lighter purples.
Brown	• Adds warmth. • Traditional. • Elegance and sophistication.
Grey	• Brings warmth and comfort. • Timeless in lighter shades. • Edgy and moderns in darker shades.
White	• Brings calming effects. • Makes room feel open and spacious.
Black	• Best in small doses. • Grounds color scheme. • Gives depth.
Metallics	• Gives instant style. • Adds durability. • Promotes excitement and creativity.

Adapted from My Move's "Room Color and How it Affects Your Mood" (Borrelli, 2021)

To facilitate safety, independence, and functionality, chair or toilet seats should contrast with floor colors so seat edges are more easily visible, similar to contrasting colors of sinks and countertops or dishes and table coverings. Conversely, high contrasting bold patterns in floor coverings should be avoided, but distinct color changes at doorways and for handrails enhances their visibility. Finally, variety in color lends a homelike feel, versus the institutional look of rooms all being painted the same drab color. In fact, allowing a resident to select the wall color for their own room helps them personalize it, and encouraging residents to work together to select paint colors or other accoutrements for public spaces increases ownership, feelings of community, and a sense of belonging.

Vision changes as part of the aging process may require three to five times as much light than young eyes (Brawley, 2006). When lighting levels are low, residents may have difficulty ambulating or engaging in meaningful leisure activities. Poor lighting also increases fall risks, which are detrimental to independence and mobility and can negatively impact quality of life. Beyond preventing these issues, when light levels are significantly increased in care communities, residents experience fewer sleep problems and sundowning behaviors among those with dementia (Brawley, 2006). Beyond adequate lighting, another concern can be glare, which is when bright light interferes with something less bright, and can cause confusion and agitation, decreased activity, and compromised safety. Some care communities have even implemented lighting systems throughout buildings that mimic natural light patterns (i.e., cycled lighting interventions) throughout the day, which may aid residents in developing a healthier circadian rhythm for better sleep and increase their participation in activities (Giggins et al., 2019) (see Exhibit 5.13).

Exhibit 5.13 Findings From the *Sleep-Wake Research Centre*
Light therapy was first developed to treat seasonal depression, but its success led to its use in other areas, including residents with dementia. Two newer studies in Swiss nursing homes illustrate how light as an "architectural treatment" is becoming popular. In one study, dynamic ceiling lighting in the day-room providing warm-white, lower intensity light in the morning and evening, and cool-white higher intensity light during the day, was compared to conventional constant lighting in care of individuals with severe dementia. Patients with higher average individual daily light exposure showed significantly longer expression of emotional pleasure, were more alert per daily observation than patients with lower daily light exposure, had higher quality of life, spent less time in bed, and went to bed later. With later sleep onset.

A second study used an LED dawn-dusk simulation (DDS) lamp at the head of the bed, for 20 residents with dementia. It was programmed for a slow naturalistic rise in light intensity in the morning and a similar, slow decline at night before sleep onset. Mood and cheerfulness upon awakening was significantly higher with the DDS, as was circadian stability (regularity of sleep-wake cycles) and ratings of quality of life.

Adapted from Center for Environmental Therapeutics' "Life and Light in a Nursing Home" (Munch, 2021)

To enhance the environment, overall light levels should be substantially raised and coupled with natural daylight. Using brighter bulbs or increasing the number of light sources raises the level of illumination. Lighter paint colors and increased lighting of walls and ceilings enhance surface brightness. Expanding the number and size of windows or using skylights will enhance natural light. In residents' rooms, using lamps in addition to ceiling mounted or traditional over-the-bed light fixtures increases ambient lighting and creates a more homelike, less institutional, feel.

Lighting levels can then easily be altered to suit individual activities and moods, leaving room for autonomy. Shielding bulbs with lamp shades or using ceiling facing light sources, like cove or pendant fixtures, reduces direct light and glare. Care centers can also install blinds, awnings, or light-shelves to bounce light toward ceilings to reduce glare from windows, buffed floors, and metal equipment.

It can be difficult to get used to the ambient noise of a residential care community. Besides the general noise of multiple care recipients and staff all sharing the space in a resident's home, there are institutional noises such as alarms or overhead paging systems that disrupt the serenity of a homelike environment. Additionally, other noises may include calling out or yelling by residents or staff, or perhaps background music that is piped throughout the building that residents cannot control. When these extraneous sounds are layered with the sounds produced by residents—televisions playing, telephones ringing, activities being conducted, and general conversations between residents, staff, and visitors—the distress of environmental noise can become problematic (Kane et al., 2004) and it may be difficult to find a peaceful, quiet place, especially for those residents who lack a private bedroom.

To address ambient noise, care communities should use technology to move away from overhead paging and auditory alarms. Additionally, changing care practices to better engage residents with loud behaviors can reduce disruptions and enhance all residents' quality of life. Providing quiet communal spaces is important, whether in a chapel, library, meditation room, or garden. Even the decision to play music in some public spaces should be done thoughtfully, since some residents may have different preferences for musical genres and others desire a music-free environment. Compromises may be necessary: some care centers utilize a rotation of musical genres (or no music) played at mealtimes or social events. Other facilities employ technology such as wireless headphones to allow those who wish to listen to music, audio books, or other aural stimulation to do so while not disrupting other residents who seek a quieter environment. Exhibit 5.14 provides helpful examples for care centers to use in improving the quality and frequency of sounds for residents.

Exhibit 5.14 Improving the Soundscape of Long-Term Care
Many sounds compete for the attention of nursing home staff members, including ringing telephones, television sets, conversations, overhead pages, elders calling for help, alarms, equipment, call bell signals, and more. All of these extraneous noises contribute to the cacophony of the environment experienced by residents and staff alike.

Some adjustments that can enhance the aural environment include:

- Eliminating overhead pages in favor of systems with individual alerts or alerts on mobile devices.
- Removing chair and bed alarms, which add to the clamor but not to reduction of falls.
- Provide adequate nursing staff trained to answer call bells promptly.

(continued)

Exhibit 5.14 (continued)
- Hold interdisciplinary meetings to identify and treat disruptive residents.
- Review the need for resident wander guards, and discontinue if possible.
- Train staff to address resident discord before it escalates.
- Provide communication systems for team members to contact each other quickly and quietly.
- Educate staff to reduce loud conversations at night, and lower television and radio volumes during quiet hours.
- Consider acoustic ceiling tiles and sound machines that play ocean sounds.
- Provide wireless headphones for residents who prefer a louder television.

The soundscape has a great impact on residents and staff and improvements can enhance the experiences of those who live and work in nursing homes.

Adapted from McKnight's Long Term Care News' "The Sounds of LTC" (Barbera, 2018)

As people get older, their metabolic rate may slow, leading to lower body heat or greater sensitivity to drafts (Wrublowsky, 2018). Temperature, like many environmental factors, often goes unnoticed when it is comfortable. However, when a resident becomes cold or too warm, it is a significant distraction to comfort and well-being. Temperatures in common areas should be set to collective residents' likings, although it may make for a warmer than usual environment for staff. To avoid drafts, ventilation systems should be designed thoughtfully, with vents set to avoid blowing air across areas where residents congregate. Ideally, residents should be able to control the temperature within their own bedroom by making thermostat adjustments, as well as opening and closing their windows.

5.2   Creating Safe and Functional Access to the Outdoors

Care recipients' well-being is improved when they have the ability to leave the confines of the walls of the care community. There is strong evidence that access to nature has positive impacts on resident physical, psychological, and behavioral health (Calkins, n.d.). Care recipients who spend more time outdoors have lower rates of depression and residents who participate in gardening and other outdoor programs have an improved mood, ability to concentrate, and patterns of sleep (see Exhibit 5.15). Residents who spend time outdoors have higher rates of Vitamin D and fewer falls (Liu, 1997), which preserves mobility and independence, and they have less stress and agitation (Calkins, n.d.). Outside spaces engage the senses and engender participation in meaningful activities (Eikelboom, 2017).

Exhibit 5.15 The Healing Power of Nature

A growing body of research has shown that nature can be a powerful tool for longevity, emotional well-being, and independence. Enjoying nature can help seniors:

- Give their immune systems a boost.
- Help relieve stress, anxiety, and depression.
- Increases energy levels.
- Improve memory and concentration.
- Reduce chronic illness and pain.
- Increase longevity.

Caregivers can help residents connect with nature by helping them:

- Go for a walk.
- Participate in gardening.
- Find time to relax outside.
- Engage in a novel outdoor activity.
- Bring the natural world inside.

Adapted from Companions for Seniors' "The Healing Power of Nature for Seniors".

Some of the biggest barriers to ensuring long-term care recipients' access to the outdoors are availability of secure outdoor spaces and concerns about safety and supervision. From a safety perspective, it is ideal for outdoor spaces to be enclosed, especially so those with cognitive impairment do not inadvertently wander off. It is also important, however, to encourage residents to be as independent as possible, allowing them direct, relatively unrestricted access to safe and secure outdoor spaces. This can be facilitated by the use of automatic or coded doors exiting to outdoor spaces with a defined boundary. The outdoor space itself must also be designed with safety in mind, including level walking surfaces, handrails, and appropriately spaced benches for resting.

For maximum benefit, several additional design elements should be considered. A covered porch can help residents' eyes adjust to outdoor lighting changes and provide a shady place to sit. Comfortable furniture, in both sunny and shady areas, arranged in conversation pods (as opposed to a row of seating) invites residents and guests to socialize. Fans or heaters should also be employed to keep outside spaces comfortable across seasons. Landscaping with trees and shrubs are enjoyable to enhance the outdoor ambience, as are water features such as a fountain (Fig. 5.8).

To attract residents to use outdoor spaces, beyond a place to sit, opportunities for engagement should be provided, such as gardening spaces, with raised planters featuring available, accessible gardening tools and supplies (Fig. 5.9). Beyond enjoying the beauty of nature or engaging in horticulture or conversation, outdoor spaces also lend themselves to activities such as morning flag-raising ceremonies,

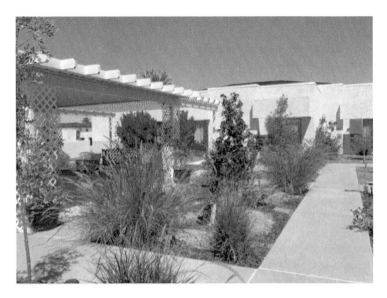

Fig. 5.8 At Veterans Homes of California in Barstow, the outdoor garden space has smooth pathways, seating pods in shaded areas, and plenty of sunshine. Many of residents senses are engaged when they spend time outside in the fresh air. Photo Credit: U.S. Department of Veterans Affairs

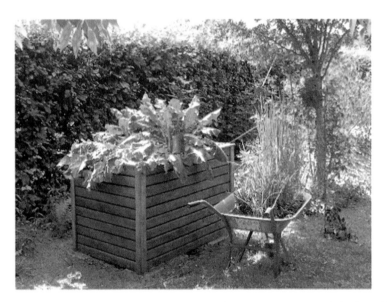

Fig. 5.9 Raised garden beds at a care community's outdoor green space are tended to by residents as part of their Life Enrichment program. Residents feel a sense of purpose when they play a role in helping to beautify their environment. Photo Credit: Ulrike Mai

picnic events, or places to play yard games. Designing outdoor spaces with multi-use in mind, and furnishing them with walking paths, group gathering spaces, and the supplies and equipment for a variety of leisure activities, makes outdoor spaces appealing to residents and increases their usage.

Even if residents are reticent to go outside, having a view of the area surrounding the care center, whether of a garden, park, busy street, or a tree, enhances their life satisfaction (Eikelboom, 2017). Buildings should be designed so residents have access to see out the window of their personal bedroom and communal spaces should have large windows with outside views, including comfortable seating from which views can be enjoyed. Some residents may enjoy observing their peers gardening or engaging in other outdoor activities, and seeing outdoor spaces being used by peers may entice a hesitant resident to venture outside. Other ways to encourage usage of outdoor spaces include having restrooms nearby, providing sunglasses and hats at doorways, and ensuring a staff member is available or nearby if assistance is needed.

5.3 Environmental Considerations for Residents with Dementia

Long-term care communities' physical environments should be built to support residents' functional abilities and quality of life by playing to their strengths while reducing demands (Cutler, 2008). Nearly 50% of long-term care recipients have dementia (Centers for Disease Control and Prevention, 2021) and most residents experience various cognitive changes as part of the normal aging process (Murman, 2015). Care recipients experiencing cognitive decline can be supported through the thoughtful design of their physical environment.

Wandering by cognitively impaired residents can be a challenging behavior to manage, but it is also an adaptive behavior for some residents seeking stimulation or self-soothing. Residents may wander less when the design elements described throughout this chapter have been employed. An example of creatively solving the issue of wandering is presented in Exhibit 5.16. Intentionally creating safe places for residents to walk and wander is also beneficial, as when residents feel access is being prevented it can lead to agitation or aggression (Wrublowsky, 2018). Supporting wandering allows for cognitive stimulation, exercise, and alleviates the burden of constant redirection from staff. It also increases feelings of comfort and satisfaction among residents with dementia (Cohen-Mansfield & Werner, 1998), and they have better moods, less anger and anxiety, and increased interest and pleasure (Wrublowsky, 2018). Designated wandering spaces, whether indoors or outdoors, should be integrated throughout common areas and activity spaces and utilize favorable stimuli along pathways.

Exhibit 5.16 Art Gallery in a Wandering Path
A permanent art gallery was created as an integral part of the "Margherita" day center for Alzheimer's disease in Fano, Italy. It is open to Margherita users and visitors as well as to all citizens. This promotes integration between the center, its users, and the city. A "Wandering Path" is quite literally that: a winding walkway that connects the entrance to the three different units that make up the center (divided according to the severity of the dementia) and to spaces for shared activities and gardens.
Adapted from Argentum's "Senior Living Innovation Series: Memory Care" (2016).

Wandering can create issues when cognitively impaired residents enter peer's rooms or handle their things uninvited, leaving the occupant feeling vulnerable or violated and experiencing emotional distress (Boonstra, 2014). Although a closed door may solve this issue, many residents prefer to stay connected to and observe others' activity by keeping their doors open and cognitively impaired residents may do better if they have a visual sightline to caregivers. Additionally, sometimes a closed door only further piques wandering residents' curiosity. Design alternatives may include using half doors, attaching a fabric or mesh "gate" that can be extended across the threshold (Wrublowsky, 2018), or even a simple dark, thick visual line painted or taped across the threshold, which may be enough to deter some wanders from entering.

Orientation and wayfinding can leave cognitively impaired residents feeling confused and agitated. Residents with dementia tend to navigate their environments with a focus on external signals, so their independence should be supported with architectural cues, especially where direction changes (Slaughter & Morgan, 2012). Their navigation is enhanced when the design is unique to discrete locations so they can independently identify and access their own bedrooms and bathroom, as well as common living spaces, like lounges and kitchens, and safe outdoor spaces. Memory boxes can be mounted outside residents' bedrooms to hold personal artifacts and, with permission, their names can be posted as well, also serving as a catalyst for conversation and relationship building (see Exhibit 5.17). Bedroom doors can be uniquely different from each other in design, color, hardware, or décor, to enhance the likelihood a resident is locating the correct room (Passini et al. 2000).

Exhibit 5.17 Ways Memory Boxes Improve the Resident Experience
- **Valuable Memory Tool**—they prompt for orientation and wayfinding and provide both a navigational aid and a calming influence.
- **Build Community**—displaying memorabilia, whether photos or objects, offers a window into a resident's life, which can prompt conversation and assist in building rapport and connectivity with both residents and staff.

(continued)

Exhibit 5.17 (continued)
- **Enhance the Residential Environment**—they are personal and sample each resident's individuality, turning a facility into a residence.

Adapted from Assisted Living Memory Boxes' "Dementia Memory Boxes: Seeing Benefits" (2019).

Residents, especially those with dementia, may pose an elopement risk. Exhibit 5.18 presents practical strategies to prevent resident elopement. Exits are challenging because they need to be easily accessible, yet not alluring to entice cognitively impaired residents to leave. Besides the danger to and agitation of the eloping resident, elopements can be disturbing to other residents, as often to prevent elopement, doors sound alarms when unauthorized exits occur, disturbing and disrupting those who live there. One strategy is to affix a panel of cloth with Velcro, to cover door hardware (Namazi et al., 1989), reducing automatic impulses to turn the knob and identification of a door as something that should be exited. Doors and nearby walls can be disguised with painted murals. Grid patterns or wide flooring stripes can serve as visual barriers but should not be used as a sole strategy. To support those who elope or have a strong urge to leave, one facility in Germany erected a bench and a bus stop sign near the front of their building (although no bus stopped there). It was a safe, attractive place for residents to sit and wait until they could be located and supported (Miller, 2011).

Exhibit 5.18 Approaches to Prevent Elopement
1. Thoroughly assess all new admissions for confusion, cognitive impairment, and history of exit-seeking.
2. Complete a thorough risk-assessment that includes asking whether the resident makes statements about wanting to go home, opens doors for no reason, displays behavior that an elopement may be forthcoming, backs their belongings, or loiters near doors.
3. Determine if family members have used successful strategies to prevent unsafe wandering or successful exiting.
4. Create secure outdoor environments free of obstructions with adequate lighting and low glare. Make sure walking surfaces and transitions are smooth.
5. Provide easy, safe, and secure access to the outdoors while maintaining control over unauthorized exiting and accompanying residents at risk of elopement when outdoors.
6. Keep items typically picked up before leaving the house (e.g., car keys, umbrella, coat) out of sight, as they may trigger wandering or elopement.
7. Develop a preventive action plan for resident at risk of elopement.

(continued)

Exhibit 5.18 (continued)

8. Evaluate the "who, what, where, and how" of an elopement incident to determine what interventions should be added or changed to prevent in the future.
9. Assess any change in condition related to exit-seeking behavior routinely.

Adapted from the State of Wisconsin's "Nursing Home Strategies to Enhance Quality of Life for Residents with Dementia" (2015).

Nostalgic memories and items from individual's past—either personal in nature or reminiscent of activities they used to enjoy, can be excellent tools for reducing agitation or other challenging behaviors among those with memory care issues. Using architectural style or design elements from the decades in which memory care residents grew up delivers a sense of familiarity. The benefit of connecting with past memories underscores the importance of residents being able to retain personal items and photos in their bedrooms, and supports the use building spaces for life skills stations, further described in the Activities and Religious Practices chapter, where residents can see and use the equipment, tools, and supplies one would use to perform these various life activities. Exhibit 5.19 shares an innovative example of creating past objects for residents in care centers to improve resident quality of life.

Exhibit 5.19 An Object From the Past
Martin Luther Care Center partnered with the University of Minnesota to assess whether creating three-dimensional (3D) printed objects could assist residents in participating in deeper reminiscing therapy by physically holding objects from their past in their hands. Several residents expressed deep joy once they were able to hold their 3D reminiscence object in their hands. Family members were highly satisfied and felt their loved ones benefited from this intervention, and among participating residents, a reduction of falls was observed along with an increase in participation in facility activities.
Adapted from "An Object From the Past" (Purdie, n.d.)

5.4 Essential Influencers

Some key stakeholders play especially important roles in helping to both structure and ensure utilization of the environment such that it maximizes residents' quality of life.

5.4.1 Social Workers

At the time of admission, social workers (or admissions directors) should encourage residents and families to help personalize care recipients' space with their own belongings and items of personal significance. They should invite family members to be a part of the move-in process, explaining options for personalization along the way. Social workers (or admissions coordinators) should also give a tour of the care center to the residents and family members if they have not already had one, and they can point out all the common areas, inside and out, that residents and families are encouraged to use for socializing and other activities. Social workers should assist residents in mitigating any roommate conflicts that may arise due to differences in lifestyle preferences, especially with respect to environmental noise and privacy concerns, and help residents to find alternative places within the care community where they can enjoy solitude. They should also help assist residents who desire to host guests, finding them spaces they can gather with friends and family outside their bedrooms, when appropriate.

5.4.2 Maintenance Personnel

Maintenance personnel can play a key role in helping residents to personalize their space. They can paint bedroom walls a color of the resident's choice prior to move-in and if residents opt to bring their own furniture, maintenance personnel can arrange to move and store any facility-owned furniture in advance of the move-in. During the move-in process they can assist in resident room personalization by moving furniture and belongings and hanging pictures on walls. Throughout the building, these staff members can ensure accommodations are in place to promote independence and provide ergonomically appropriate furniture and toileting equipment to meet each resident's unique needs. They are also instrumental in keeping the environment in good repair and promptly completing any necessary repairs, such as replacing flickering or burned-out light bulbs, mopping up liquid spills, and repairing cracked or uneven flooring to ensure resident safety and comfort.

5.4.3 Nursing and Direct Care Staff

Beyond encouraging personalization of their room, a key role for nursing and direct care staff is ensuring environmental comfortability. This can be done by advocating for environmental changes to outdated bathing environments and personally, by ensuring residents are comfortable in their rooms. For example, direct care staff can assist residents in adjusting the temperature, offering them an extra blanket, or ensuring they have comfortable seating and can see out the window if that is their preference. Some care centers have even implemented new positions, sometimes titled "hospitality aides," to focus exclusively on meeting comfort needs of care recipients; making rounds of the facility to offer water, snacks, books, or extra pillows; transportation to a new location; or anything else that might enhance their comfort.

5.4.4   Activities Director

In care communities with a variety of indoor and outdoor communal spaces available, the activities director must establish programming to maximize their use and ensure that such spaces are also stocked with appropriate equipment and supplies to facilitate resident engagement. For example, if communal kitchen space is available, they should offer cooking or baking activities, start a gardening club if outside spaces are secured, or host a movie night if a theatre or multipurpose space has a large screen. In common areas designed for socialization, providing activities such as large print books, word finds, puzzles, cards, and games will ensure that residents feel comfortable using such spaces both for conversation and activities with peers, but also so they can participate in solo activities (e.g., reading, crossword puzzles) in a social environment, to promote connectedness within the care community.

5.4.5   Dining Staff

Environmentally, regardless of the dining programs in place, dining staff should work to deinstitutionalize the spaces and ambiance used for meal service. This may include transferring residents who use wheelchairs into comfortable chairs during the dining experience, and giving additional considerations to décors, such as table linens, centerpieces, tableware, presentation of food, and dress and demeanor of serving staff.

References

Andrade, C., Lima, M., Devlin, A., & Hernández, B. (2016). Is it the place or the people? Disentangling the effects of hospitals' physical and social environments on Well-being. *Environment and Behavior, 48*(2), 299–323. https://doi.org/10.1177/0013916514536182

Argentum. (2016). *Senior living innovation series: Memory care*. https://www.argentum.org/images/alfa/PDFs/EMR/EMR%20MC.pdf

Assisted Living Memory Boxes. (2019, October 14). *Dementia memory boxes: Seeing benefits*. https://assistedlivingmemoryboxes.com/blog/index.php/2019/10/14/the-benefits-of-dementia-memory-boxes/.

Barbera, E. F. (2018, October 9). *The sounds of LTC*. McKnight's Long-Term Care News. https://www.mcknights.com/blogs/the-world-according-to-dr-el/the-sounds-of-ltc/.

Barrick, A., Rader, J., Hoeffer, B., Sloane, P., & Biddle, S. (2008). *Bathing without a Battle: Person-directed Care of Individuals with dementia*. Springer.

Boonstra, N. (2014). *Privacy in personal care homes in Winnipeg, Manitoba as experienced by residents*. Thesis, Manitoba, Winnipeg, Canada. Retrieved from https://mspace.lib.umanitoba.ca/xmlui/bitstream/handle/1993/23920/Privacy%20in%20personal%20care%20homes%20in%20Winnipeg%20Manitoba%20as%20experienced%20by%20residents.pdf?sequence=5&isAllowed=y.

Borrelli, L. (2021, February 9). *Room color and how it affects your mood.* My Move. https://www.mymove.com/home-inspiration/decoration-design-ideas/room-color-and-how-it-affects-your-mood/.

Bowman, C. (2008). The environmental side of the culture change movement: Identifying barriers and potential solutions to furthering innovation in nursing homes. *Creating Home in the nursing Home: A National Symposium on culture change and the environment requirements* (pp. 1–93). Center for Medicare and Medicaid Services & Edu-Catering. Retrieved from https://www.pioneernetwork.net/wp-content/uploads/2016/10/The-Environmental-Side-of-the-Culture-Change-Movement-Symposium-Background-Paper-1.pdf

Brawley, E. (1997). *Designing for Alzheimer's disease: Strategies for better care environments.* John Wiley and Sons.

Brawley, E. (2006). *Design innovations for aging and Alzheimer's: Creating caring environments.* John Wiley & Sons.

Calkins, M. (n.d.). *Designing gardens to attract activity.* Pioneer Network. Retrieved from Pioneer Network: https://www.pioneernetwork.net/resource-categories/physical-environment/

Calkins, M., & Cassella, C. (2007). Exploring the cost and value of private versus shared bedrooms in nursing homes. *The Gerontologist, 47*(2), 169–183.

Centers for Disease Control and Prevention. (2021, March 1). National Center for Health Statistics. Retrieved from Alzheimer Disease: https://www.cdc.gov/nchs/fastats/alzheimers.htm.

Cohen-Mansfield, J., & Werner, P. (1998). The effects of an enhanced environment on nursing home residents who pace. *The Gerontologist, 38*(2), 199–208.

Cutler, L. (2008). Nothing is traditional about environments in a traditional nursing Home: Nursing homes as places to live now and In the future. *Creating home in the nursing home: A national symposium on culture change and the environmental requirements* (pp. 1–29). Centers for Medicare and Medicaid Services. Retrieved from https://www.pioneernetwork.net/wp-content/uploads/2016/10/Nothing-is-Traditional-about-Environments-Paper.pdf

Eikelboom, H. V. (2017). Architectural factors influencing the sense of home in nursing homes: An operationalization for practice. *Frontiers of Architectural Research, 6,* 111–122. https://doi.org/10.1016/j.foar.2017.02.004

Falk, H., Wijk, H., Persson, L., & Falk, K. (2013). A sense of home in residential care. *Scandinavian Journal of Caring Sciences, 27,* 999–1009.

Giggins, O. M., Doyle, J., Hogan, K., & George, M. (2019). The impact of a cycled lighting intervention on nursing home residents: A pilot study. *Gerontology and Geriatric Medicine, 5,* 2333721419897453. https://doi.org/10.1177/2333721419897453

Harrar, S., Eaton, J. & Meyer, H. (2021, January 13). *10 Steps to reform and improve nursing homes.* AARP. https://www.aarp.org/caregiving/health/info-2021/steps-to-improve-nursing-homes.html

Holm, C. (n.d.). *How cats enhance a nursing Home setting.* Fear Free Pets. https://fearfreepets.com/how-cats-enhance-a-nursing-home-setting/

Jarrett, C. (2013). The psychology of stuff and things. *The Psychologist, 26*(8), 560–562. https://thepsychologist.bps.org.uk/volume-26/edition-8/psychology-stuff-and-things

Johs-Artisensi, J., Hansen, K., & Olson, D. (2020). Qualitative analyses of nursing home residents' quality of life from multiple stakeholders' perspectives. *Quality of Life Research, 29*(5), 1229–1238. https://doi.org/10.1007/s11136-019-02395-3

Johs-Artisensi, J., Hansen, K., & Olson, D. C. (2021). Leadership perceptions and practices of hospitality in senior care. *Journal of Applied Gerontology, 40*(6), 598–597. https://doi.org/10.1177/0733464820923903

Kane, R., Kane, R., Bershadsky, B., Cutler, L., Giles, K., Liu, J., ... Zhang, L. (2004). *Measures, indicators.* Centers for Medicare and Medicaid Services.

Kane, R., Kling, K., Bershadsky, B., Kane, R., Giles, K., Degenholtz, H., ... Cutler, L. (2003). Quality of life measures for nursing Home residents. *The Journals of Gerontology: Series A, 58*(3), M240–M248. https://doi.org/10.1093/gerona/58.3.M240

Koren, M. (2010, February). Person-centered care for nursing Home residents: The culture-change movement. *Health Affairs, 29*(2), 312–317.

Liu, B. (1997). Seasonal prevalence of vitamin D deficiency in institutionalized older adults. *Journal of the American Geriatrics Society, 45*(5), 598–603.

Miller, L. (2011). *A bus to nowhere* [Recorded by L. Miller]. Radiolab Podcast (Season 9, Episode 4). Retrieved from https://www.wnycstudios.org/podcasts/radiolab/segments/121385-bus-nowhere

Munch, M. (2021). *Life and light in a nursing home.* Center for Environmental Therapeutics'. https://cet.org/life-and-light-in-a-nursing-home/.

Murman, D. (2015). The impact of age on cognition. *Seminars in Hearing, 36*(3), 111–121. https://doi.org/10.1055/s-0035-1555115

Namazi, K. H., Rosner, T. T., & Calkins, M. P. (1989). Visual barriers to prevent ambulatory Alzheim-er's patients from exiting through an emergency door. *The Gerontologist, 29*(5), 699–702.

Passini, R., Pigot, H., Rainville, C., & Tetreault, M. H. (2000). Wayfinding in a nursing home for advanced dementia of the Alzheimer's type. *Environment and Behavior, 32*(5), 684–710.

Pioneer Network. (2011). *A guide to better care options for an aging America.* The Picker Institute. Retrieved from https://www.pioneernetwork.net/wp-content/uploads/2016/10/Creating-Home-Consumer-Guide.pdf.

Purdie, C. (n.d.). *An object from the past.* University of Wisconsin - Eau Claire. https://www.uwec.edu/files/634/Object-from-the-Past-Purdie.pdf

Rijnaard, M. V. (2016). The factors influencing the sense of home in nursing homes: A systematic review from the perspective of residents. *Journal of Aging Research*, Epub. https://doi.org/10.1155/2016/6143645.

Salonena, H., Lahtinena, M., Lappalainena, S., Nevalac, N., Knibbs, L., Morawska, L., & Reijulaf, K. (2013). Physical characteristics of the indoor environment that affect health and Well-being in healthcare facilities: A review. *Intelligent Buildings International, 5*(1), 3–25. https://doi.org/10.1080/17508975.2013.764838

Selfhelp Home. (2016). *Hotel like suites are the new nursing home.* https://selfhelphome.org/hotel-like-suites-are-the-new-nursing-home/.

Shields, S. N. (2006). *In pursuit of the sunbeam: A practical guide to transformation from institution to household.* Action Pact Press.

Slaughter, S., & Morgan, D. (2012). Functional outcomes of nursing Home residents in relation to features of the environment: Validity of the professional environmental assessment protocol. *Journal of the American Medical Directors Association, 13*(5), e1–e7. https://doi.org/10.1016/j.jamda.2012.01.003

Social Care Institute for Excellence. (n.d.). *Activities for people with dementia based around food.* https://www.scie.org.uk/dementia/living-with-dementia/eating-well/activities-around-food.asp

Stempak, N. (2017, November 21). *Personalized doors help residents with dementia to find their way.* i Advance Senior Care. https://www.iadvanceseniorcare.com/personalized-doors-help-residents-with-dementia-to-find-their-way/

The Green House Project. (n.d.). *The green house project: Revolutionizing care to empower lives.* Retrieved from https://thegreenhouseproject.org/

Verbeek, H. (2016). Small-scale, homelike care in nursing homes. In N. A. Pachana (Ed.), *Encyclopedia of geropsychology.* Springer. https://doi.org/10.1007/978-981-287-082-7_91

Wolfe, M. (1978). Childhood and privacy. In I. Altman & J. F. Wohlwill (Eds.), *Children and the environment. Human behavior and environment (advances in theory and research)* (Vol. 3, pp. 175–222). Springer. https://doi.org/10.1007/978-1-4684-3405-7_6

Wrublowsky, R. (2018). *Design guide for long-term care homes.* MMP Architects. Retrieved from https://www.fgiguidelines.org/wp-content/uploads/2018/03/MMP_DesignGuideLongTermCareHomes_2018.01.pdf.

Yildirim, K., Akalin-Baskaya, A., & Hidayetoglu, M. (2007). Effects of indoor color on mood and cognitive performance. *Building and Environment, 42*(9), 3233–3240. https://doi.org/10.1016/j.buildenv.2006.07.037

Chapter 6
Food and Dining

Food, glorious food! What is there more handsome? Gulped, swallowed, or chewed – Still worth a king's ransom! – "Food, Glorious Food" from Oliver

Abstract When interviewing long-term care residents on aspects of their daily lives that have the greatest impact, food—and dining services, overall—often ranks at the very top of the list. The content in this chapter discusses food preparation, dining preferences, selection at meal times, the dining experience, and delivery of meals in long-term care settings. The importance of nutrition and hydration for older adults, as part of carefully crafted menus and meals, is also covered. Attention is carefully paid to distinguishing current approaches in culinary services from more resident-focused, resident-driven best practices, such as those practice which align with culture change principles for individualization and those which are thoughtfully tailored to resident preferences. In addition to the selection of dietary items, the setting in which meals are served (e.g., shifts away from gargantuan dining halls to a more restaurant-styled atmosphere) will be discussed, as well as different hospitality-centered nomenclature for staff (e.g., "servers" rather than the traditional "dietary aide"). Resident choice and autonomy, including meal preferences, are a predominant focus of this domain that substantially affects quality of life.

Keywords Food · Dining services · Nutrition · Hydration · Menus · Food preparation · Aging changes with food · Food service · Meal times · Food consumption · Quality of meals · Culinary services · Hospitality · Culture change · Dietary services · Individualized meals · Modified diets · Dining environment · Farm to table · Role of staff

From anecdotal stories to evidence-based research, one of the primary factors that can significantly influence quality of life for residents in long-term care communities is food and the dining experience. Several studies have included food and the dining experience as an essential element relative to overall quality of life in care centers (e.g., R. L. Kane et al., 2005). While some studies focus on the nutritional value of food intake and the prevention of malnutrition—important, indeed, to consider for resident health—the ability to have a pleasurable meal experience and have some determination in the meal choice itself gives residents a sense of control over one important aspect of life in long-term care and senior living settings.

As far back as 2008, researchers predicted the increase in resident desire for improved food choices and delivery options for long-term and residential care settings (Robinson & Gallagher, 2008). The Danish Food Administration, for example, has recommended that facilities have a food and meal policy that encompasses the quality of food, the meal itself, and the dining environment (Kuosma et al., 2008). In care settings that serve older adults with physical impairments, the food experience may need to be modified, yet should remain a pleasurable and enjoyable experience to enhance and promote optimal quality of life.

A recent study, surveying providers in US nursing homes, identified four main themes related to food and the dining experience in long-term care communities: (a) compliance with regulations, budgetary concerns, and food quality were rated as significant challenges for resident dining experiences; (b) resident satisfaction is driven primarily by the quality and taste of food provided, as well as the variety of menu options; (c) the priority for providers in long-term care settings is to improve food quality and taste even more, which is hampered by staffing shortages; and (d) providers continue to innovate in ways that improve clinical care outcomes and hospitality practices for dining service (Skilled Nursing News, 2021).

The connection between proper nutrition and hydration and its subsequent effect on resident quality of life has been well studied. Improved physical outcomes and overall health of residents, supported by ample and appropriate nutrition and hydration, can assure optimal resident health and ability to complete daily tasks (Amarantos et al., 2001), even in the presence of an illness that may impair one's abilities. Malnutrition (and inadequate hydration) has been shown to be linked with functional impairment, which is even more pronounced for residents with cognitive impairments (Stange et al., 2013; Verbrugghe et al., 2013). With appropriate nutrition (including the use of supplements, as needed), residents' cognitive function is supported and, in some cases, has been hypothesized to improve (Stange et al., 2013). This has the potential to lead to greater resident autonomy and independence in care settings through the prevention of both physical and cognitive functional declines (Fig. 6.1).

6.1 Aging Changes that Affect Food Consumption

There are many factors that can affect an older adult's ability to enjoy a meal which are inherent in the aging process. Over time, as part of the normal aging process, appetite responses can change and, beyond that, one's food intake can be affected by certain mood and behavioral disorders (Desai et al., 2007) (see Exhibit 6.1). With pathologic aging, various health conditions can present swallowing disorders that may affect an older adult's ability to eat certain foods, and there can be other physical

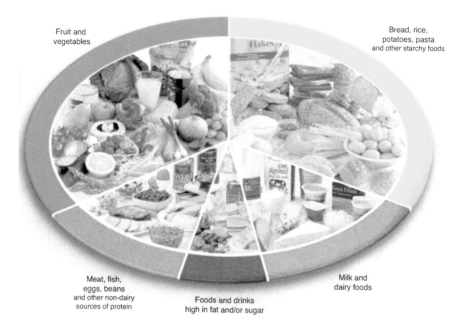

Fruit and
vegetables

Bread, rice,
potatoes, pasta
and other starchy foods

Meat, fish,
eggs, beans
and other non-dairy
sources of protein

Foods and drinks
high in fat and/or sugar

Milk and
dairy foods

Fig. 6.1 Diagram of "The Eatwell Plate" which recommends appropriate portions of various food groups to ensure proper nutritional intake for nursing home and care center residents from meals and snacks provided. This guide was provided in the 2014 "Nutritional Guidelines and Menu Checklist for Residential and Nursing Homes," funded through the Public Health Agency in Belfast, Northern Ireland. The guide also provides useful appendices for care centers to utilize, including assistance to assure nutritional value in general menus, appropriate portion sizes, food fortification with regular meal items, and sample "finger food" ideas for snacks (Harper et al., 2014)

conditions that can prevent self-feeding (e.g., hand tremors that affect one's ability to hold and use silverware). Some medications can affect the resident's taste for different foods, altering what otherwise would have been an enjoyable meal. Some residents develop a form of dementia (e.g., Alzheimer's disease) or a neurocognitive disorder that can impair the ability to feed oneself during meals. If residents experience weight loss or malnutrition, that has been shown to be associated with greater morbidity (i.e., new chronic conditions or exacerbation of existing chronic conditions) and mortality (Desai et al., 2007). While quality of care is always important to consider, the negative effects of poor nutrition and hydration has the distinct potential to negatively affect resident quality of life.

Exhibit 6.1 The "Seven Ages of Appetite"
First Decade (ages 0–10)

- Rapid growth and dietary behaviors established.
- Particularity of certain food choices determined by child.
- Development of portion size expectations occurs.

Second Decade (ages 10–20)

- Growth in appetite and stature.
- Formative period determining food habits throughout life.
- Potential to suffer from nutritional deficiencies.

Third Decade (ages 20–30)

- Lifestyle changes may affect food behaviors.
- Potential accumulation of body fat due to offset between food consumption and energy needs.
- Development of sense of satiety to prevent overeating.

Fourth Decade (ages 30–40)

- Increased stress changes appetite and eating patterns for many adults.
- Personality traits (e.g., perfectionism, conscientiousness) may mediate stress and affect eating behavior.
- Promotion of healthy behaviors important.

Fifth Decade (ages 40–50)

- Dietary changes and nutritional needs may change to promote better health and decreased mortality, especially for those engaging in health-risk behaviors (e.g., smoking, excessive alcohol use, poor diets).

Sixth Decade (ages 50–60)

- Decrease in muscle mass (i.e., sarcopenia) and reduction in physical activities.
- Importance of maintaining healthy, varied diet (including proper levels of protein).

Seventh Decade (ages 60 and older)

- Adequate nutrition even more important, as well as emphasizing the importance of social interactions during meals.
- Importance to have healthy body weight or to be slightly overweight (protective factor).
- Effects of aging (e.g., swallowing problems, dental issues, reduced sense of taste or smell) must be addressed to ensure meal experience is enjoyable.

Adapted from BBC's 100 Year Life "How Your Age Affects Your Appetite" (Johnstone, 2018).

If a resident does not experience proper food and nutrition intake, malnutrition may result and create the potential to aggravate any current chronic conditions (Divert et al., 2015), which can decrease resident quality of life in many ways. Some example signs and effects of malnutrition are presented in Exhibit 6.2. Both the physical dining experience and the social nature of dining itself can increase a resident's food intake and their enjoyment of a particular meal, and this is true even for residents with mild cognitive impairment or more pronounced cognitive decline. Given the impaired health of many residents in care settings and the reduced ability to self-perform activities of daily living (including the ability to feed oneself), the ability to ingest food and enjoy the experience becomes a paramount concern for health-related factors, but food and the dining experience also significantly contribute to residents' quality of life, as well.

Exhibit 6.2 Signs and Effects of Malnutrition in Long-Term Care Residents

Potential causes of malnutrition:

- Dental issues.
- Chronic illnesses.
- Medications that interfere with nutrient absorption.
- Recent hospitalizations.
- Diminished taste or smell.
- Abdominal or gastrointestinal issues (e.g., pain, bloating).

Effects of malnutrition:

- Weight loss.
- Weakness and fatigue.
- Dental deterioration.
- Yellowing of the skin.
- White fingernails.
- Pressure sores or ulcers.
- Reduced quality of life.

Adapted from the Nursing Home Abuse Center's "Malnutrition from Nursing Home Neglect" (2021).

6.2 Quality of Food and Menu Options

In the United States, significant changes to resident rights and resident quality of life were implemented in 1987 as part of the sweeping Omnibus Reconciliation and Budget Act (OBRA) focused on nursing home reform. One of the policies under OBRA 1987 was to require nursing homes and care centers to use cooked and prepared food, such as what is normally served to residents at meal times, before they turn to food-alternatives (e.g., supplements) for residents in their care. This had (and has, to this day) the very real effect of improving residents' dining experiences and the amount of food consumed, which can also decrease a facility's expenses related to food alternatives via supplements that are often more expensive.

Importantly, it may be beneficial to enhance the dining experience at focused times during the resident's day. One study noted that "breakfast represents the meal with the least variation both in nutrients delivered and intakes achieved" (Young et al., 2001). While the main meal times (i.e., breakfast, lunch, dinner) are obvious targets for nutritional intake, some residents may not consume as many calories and nutrients during those meals and may instead prefer snacks later in the afternoon or before bedtime. Giving residents the ability to alter their food intake based on their preferences largely aligns with crafting a more homelike environment, and it has the distinct potential to both increase quality of life and decrease the potential for malnutrition.

In select care centers, residents have been directly involved in crafting menu selections and in planning meals. Such involvement of residents allows a facility to tailor food provided, the recipes used, and the overall meal environment to its residents' preferences and enhance the dining experience. Some care centers have incorporated food brought in from family members, too, as depicted in Exhibit 6.3. Indeed, in a study evaluating nursing homes in France, the involvement of residents in selecting recipes for food preparation enhanced residents' sensory expectations and increased satisfaction with meals provided (Van Wymelbeke et al., 2020). Residents can be asked to form an advisory committee and work directly with the dietician or food service director in a care community to have ownership and autonomy in planning menus, ingredients used in meal preparation, and the time and delivery method for meals.

Exhibit 6.3 Food from Whom?

In the United States, the federal regulations from the Centers for Medicare and Medicaid Services (CMS) provide stringent guidelines for care centers (e.g., nursing homes, skilled nursing facilities) on where they may procure food, including only those sources approved by federal, state, or local authorities.

The guidelines were clarified in 2009 to note that food may be provided to residents by family members, friends, visitors, or resident guests. While the care center is required to help the resident understand safe food practices, they may also assist family or friends in preparing food safely for the resident (e.g., not heating food too much such that the resident's mouth could be burned).

Such practices are part of necessary culture change in care communities, but are also enforced under CMS' interpretation of the OBRA legislative changes related to resident self determination and participation. Having the ability to supplement the food at one's care center with family favorites or recipes prepared according to family traditions can enhance a resident's

(continued)

Exhibit 6.3 (continued)
experience and may also promote family visitation, adding value to the meal experience with social interaction.

Adapted from CMS' memorandum on "Nursing Home Requirements for Food Procurement, Self Determination, and Participation (CMS, 2009).

In certain locations, restaurants have benefited greatly from the "farm to table" concept, driving increased consumer demand and business with more locally sourced options on the menu. So, too, the concept eventually found its way into long-term care settings (McColl, 2015). Some care centers have partnered with local elementary schools or nearby universities to grow and harvest crops that can be included in menu selections, while other facilities have used land owned by religious organizations in the area (e.g., Milwaukee Catholic Home, 2020) (see Exhibit 6.4). Depending on how the program is structured, some care facilities have even included residents in the gardening, growing, and harvesting processes as activities to engage and stimulate individuals.

Exhibit 6.4 Clare Gardens at the Milwaukee Catholic Home
The Clare Gardens is a "sustainable, organic farm-to-table program" made possible through a partnership between the care center and the Franciscan Friars of the Assumption BVM Province. Following that partnership, the Milwaukee Catholic Home established a more permanent farm as part of the Catholic Ecology Center, totaling around 18 acres.

Beyond growing vegetables and other food items utilized in the menu creation and food preparation at the care center, the new Clare Gardens also houses an orchard producing perennial fruits and bee hives, while providing a site to compost food to be more environmentally sustainable.

The fresh vegetables and fruits are an excellent addition to the other menu items provided by the Culinary Director at the Milwaukee Catholic Home. However, the site goes even further to provide educational and social experiences for residents at the Clare Gardens that are intergenerational with community members and local university students. The added value of social experiences can enhance the dining experience and build bonds with community partners, as well.

Milwaukee Catholic Home, Clare Gardens (2021).

6.3   Modified Diets and Changes to Food Preparation for Resident Health Conditions

In 2013, the National Institutes of Health in the United States noted that the prevalence of dysphagia (i.e., swallowing difficulties) was higher for residents living in nursing homes and assisted living center than their community-dwelling counterparts, with approximately 40%–60% of residents having some form of an eating difficulty. Residents with dysphagia and other difficulties eating are more prone to having a negative dining experience and may suffer from poor nutrition as a result. One study from Norway documented inconsistencies in how food is modified and residents are served when swallowing difficulties are observed, though prevalent practices included liquid and food modification to aid residents (Engh & Speyer, 2020) (Fig. 6.2). Other earlier studies have noted the importance of modifying the dining environment, decreasing the amount of distractions (e.g., extraneous sounds, music), and assuring personalized attention to residents during the dining process when dysphagia or swallowing disorders may be present, including for residents with dementia (O'Loughlin & Shanley, 1998; Watson, 1993; Hotaling, 1990).

When swallowing disorders are diagnosed, a common food modification prescribed as part of the care planning process is to alter the resident's diet using puréed or blended foods, sometimes referred to as a "texture-modified" diet. Other approaches utilize thickening liquids and, for residents with more severe conditions, feeding tubes or intravenous feeding may become necessary at some point. All of these modifications have the potential to decrease resident satisfaction with meals

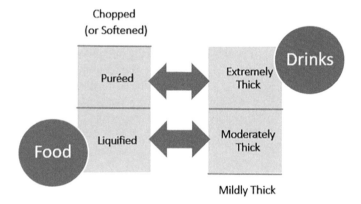

Fig. 6.2 Adapted from "Creation and Initial Validation of the International Dysphagia Diet Standardisation Initiative (IDDSI) Functional Diet Scale" (Steele, Namasivayam-MacDonald, Guida, Hanson, Lam, & Riquelme, 2018). The IDDSI scale was created and validated by Steele and colleagues using a study that showed strong validity across multiple measures and raters from 29 countries, who responded consistently to the scale. Study results indicated that the scale could be used "reliably by clinicians to capture diet texture restriction and progression in people with dysphagia." Where modified foods may not be desired by the resident, a thickened liquid might be more palatable to substitute for appropriate nutritional intake

and the dining experience but pose less risk to residents of food accidentally entering the airway while eating. Beyond modifying food options to a puréed or blended form, the American Medical Directors Association (2010) clinical practice guidelines recommend providing foods that promote "comfortable chewing and swallowing" and note that if residents refuse to consume pureed foods, other items should be offered that have a similar consistency, such as "mashed potatoes, puddings, yogurt…and finely chopped food." Regulations in the United States from the Centers for Medicare and Medicaid Services (CMS) require that any food and beverages offered to residents be "palatable, attractive, and at a safe and appetizing temperature," including any modified diets to accommodate a swallowing disorder. Even if residents need an altered consistency diet, it is important to ensure the food is presented in as normal a way as possible, including the use of food molds to imitate non-modified food and preserve dignity in the dining process for residents who may be embarrassed by this alteration.

Some residents, including those with cognitive decline, may need assistance at meal times. However, with staff properly trained in feeding assistance, residents had improved outcomes related to weight loss, body mass index (BMI), and food and fluid intake (Simmons et al., 2008), which, as previously noted, can improve quality of life as residents receive proper nutrition and hydration during their stay in a care center. This also included residents who had moderate to severe cognitive decline. When referring to residents who need assistance with meals, some nomenclature that has been used in the past in care centers includes the term "feeders" for such residents. With improved education and training for caregivers, and a culture shift within care centers to become more homelike and resident-centered, more acceptable terms have come to prominence that preserve and promote resident dignity, such as "resident who needs assistance" and "dining assistance" instead.

6.4 Improving the Dining Experience

Nursing homes and assisted living centers in numerous countries (e.g., the United States, Canada, France) have taken on the task of transforming the dining experience from a large congregate, dining hall meal, akin to a gargantuan cafeteria, to one delivered in smaller dining areas with a more homelike environment, to enhance the dining experience itself. Important in the dining transformation is the implementation of resident choice and autonomy as to when one eats, what one eats, and some direction as to how or with whom the resident dines for a meal, providing greater choice for residents in the process (Divert et al., 2015). Such changes align with the broader culture change movement, to make care more homelike rather than feeling institutional in design. Some studies have noted that food intake by residents can be positively affected by "improved plate presentation, temperature, food choice at the time of service, and portion size flexibility" (Desai et al., 2007). Optimal experiences for resident meal times should focus on resident independence, to the degree possible, while providing a setting that enhances self-esteem and gives residents a "nourishing, pleasant meal" (Speroff et al., 2005).

Other studies have noted the importance of socialization during dining processes as an essential component to prevent malnutrition and enhance the overall meal experience (Dunn & Moore, 2016; MacIntosh et al., 1989). In the United Kingdom, nursing home standards emphasize "the importance of the social aspect of dining, including the provision of an 'unhurried' social environment" (Dunn & Moore, 2016). In moving away from large dining halls to a more personalized, homelike dining environment, residents often have regular tablemates or fellow residents who commonly dine together in the same area, where they can socialize and build relationships with others in the care center and have a sense of community over a shared meal.

The dining experience itself can sometimes be one of regulatory requirement, whereby meals are prepared and served to ensure compliance with governmental regulations and less attention is paid to residents' preferences. This practice is often focused on events that occur during more precise, traditional meal times (e.g., breakfast in the morning, lunch around noon, dinner in the evening). One study noted that some Canadian nursing home processes related to meal service were fairly regimented to ensure compliance with existing regulations, although staff noted they didn't enjoy forcing residents to wake before they wished so they could eat at a proscribed time (Lowndes et al., 2015). Such has been the experience in some United States nursing homes, as well, where creative food delivery practices (e.g., setting up a breakfast station in a smaller dining area with a chef who prepares individualized meals when residents are ready to eat) designed to cater to and exceed resident wishes are more difficult to achieve under existing federal guidelines from CMS (Fig. 6.3).

In serving multiple residents who may wish to have very different schedules, food and dining service experiences have gradually transformed over time in many places to be a more flexibly timed option. Some care centers have created a la carte breakfast stations that remain open for several hours, so residents can dine when they wish to. The aromas and smells of meals cooked and served closer to the actual dining spaces, reminiscent of cooking meals at home with family members, have the potential to attract residents who may be more inclined to remain in their rooms. There are other facilities which provide snacks at various times throughout the day, in case a resident doesn't eat a full meal at a proscribed time and requires or desires sustenance later. Additionally, while sanitary food storage and serving conditions are certainly important, flexibility to allow individualized dining practices to occur should also be paramount in efforts to enhance resident quality of life.

Another methodology employed by some care centers is to have staff members (e.g., certified nurse aides, dietary aides, nursing home administrator) dine with the residents, at least on occasion (Fig. 6.4). In doing so, the goal is to promote socialization and an enjoyable meal experience which, as noted above, has been shown to promote even more food intake and increased quality of life. Such an approach has the effect of making a residential care center feel less institutionalized for residents, while still allowing staff members to assist those residents who may

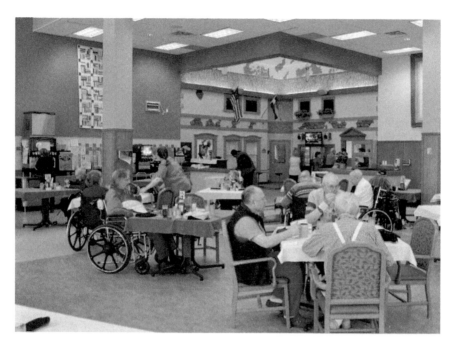

Fig. 6.3 The dining area at the Spanish Peaks Regional Health Center and Veterans Community Living Center in Colorado was created to emulate an "Italian Village" theme. There is a central gathering area with various amenities nearby the Mountain View Dining Hall, which offers food and beverages offered to resident veterans throughout the day, with staff members available at all times to help residents when they wish to have a bite to eat

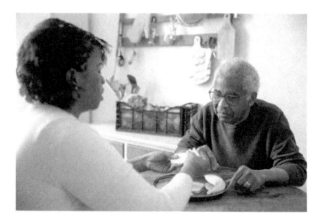

Fig. 6.4 Having staff members engage with residents during meal times is a strategy that can enhance the dining experience for the resident, but also can build a stronger bond between caregiver and care recipient. Staff members sharing a meal gives greater opportunity to learn about residents, their experiences accumulated over a lifetime, and better informs staff efforts to continually individualize aspects of care to improve resident quality of life. Photo Credit: Kampus Production

need help when dining. The relationships that dietary aides and other caregivers have with residents have been shown to significantly contribute to a positive meal experience—so much so, in some cases, that at times residents have to be encouraged to eat more because they spend significant time talking with their caregiver dining guest. "Knowing the elder, their choices, their preferences, and their daily pleasures in dining results in service that encourages optimal intake" (Bowman, 2010). Additionally, better knowledge of the resident and his or her preferences can help a dietary aide or nurse aide know which foods might entice the resident to eat and ensure proper food intake and hydration (Bowman, 2010). This can also increase staff satisfaction, as many wish to get to know the residents better while sharing a meal and having an engaging conversation. Unfortunately, prevalent staffing shortages that exist in long-term care settings across the globe—which have only worsened over time—hamper the ability of caregivers to spend extended dining time at tables with residents for socialization. With fewer staff available to accomplish the necessary daily tasks of operating care centers, the requirements of staff members only serving and assisting a set number of residents has become an utterly impractical task, as documented in several studies from various countries, let alone the additional time staff would like to spend with the residents to socialize and enhance their quality of life and meal experience.

There are multiple approaches care communities can take if they desire to create an enhanced dining experience and shift away from the medical model of providing care and services. The following practices implemented in care communities offer residents greater choice and direction in their meal selection, which can promote enhanced satisfaction with meals and increased quality of life. Some facilities have utilized a restaurant-style approach, where staff members function more like servers. Terminology such as "servers" or "waiters" is used to imitate a restaurant ambiance (rather than using "dietary aide" or something similar), and the tables look more like what one would see when dining out in public. There may be an expanded menu available for residents to select their meal from, and this approach often uses extended dining times to better cater to residents. Some facilities have involved residents in the dining process (e.g., assisting with setting tables, designing decorative centerpieces) to enhance resident participation and increase satisfaction. Other care centers have modified the restaurant approach and use a buffet service, where residents can select from items and create their own plates based on individual preferences (Fig. 6.5). For smaller long-term care communities, such as in Green House homes that serve fewer residents (Green House Project, 2021), a more family-style dining experience can be achieved. In such a model, residents with culinary prowess can cook meals alongside staff members and food can be served at a larger table that everyone sits around to dine together. Indeed, implementing a family-style dining approach improved resident quality of life and the body weight for residents in Dutch nursing homes, including for those residents with physical impairments necessitating assistance with bathing, dressing, and transferring (Nijs et al., 2006). Lastly, some care communities offer "happy hours" to their residents, either via a mobile cart or in select locations within the building. Some facilities have even built a bar and lounge area for this purpose—for alcoholic beverages to be served and to

Fig. 6.5 Thanksgiving dinners, served in a more buffet style in nursing homes and care centers for residents, can bring back fond memories of large family meals during holidays celebrated together. Many care centers also extend invitations to family members to join their loved ones for a nominal fee, to promote engagement of families and increase socialization of residents during meals and at special times of the year. Photo Credit: Brykmantra

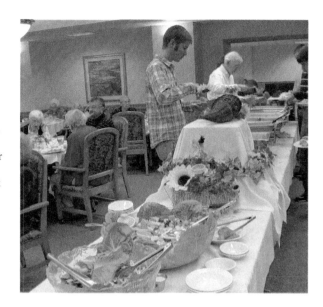

replicate an enjoyable activity that residents may have participated in prior to living at the care center.

In most cases, residents are encouraged and supported to join meal times with other residents or even staff members. However, due to physical impairment or infection control measures, some residents may need to receive meals in their rooms. Care centers have the ability to transform even a solitary dining experience for residents by making it seem comparable to what one might find when staying in a hotel on vacation. Some facilities have even utilized in-room technology, like smart televisions or tablet devices, that allow residents to order food from bed, utilizing the same menus available to residents dining in communal areas.

6.5   The Dining Environment

Several studies have articulated the importance of the dining environment itself, in addition to food quality or dining service practices, as an essential component of resident meal experiences. Overall considerations regarding the environment in care settings are covered in more detail in the Environment and Surroundings chapter. The choice of wall color, which cups and plates are used, the elimination of bibs and large serving trays, and even the use of cloth napkins (rather than disposable paper napkins) as part of an overall ambiance can significantly enhance the resident dining experience.

When thinking about an optimal dining environment for residents, something as simple as the dining room layout can enhance meal experiences, just through the ease of navigating from the hallway to their chosen table (Speroff et al., 2005).

Several studies have noted the importance of using tablecloths to "hide" a table that may be designed specifically for a facility providing care rather than one found in a gourmet restaurant. Another study of Belgian nursing homes assessed the dining environment based on (a) whether the setting was pleasant; (b) the desire to eat in the specific dining room; (c) the staff members who served residents; (d) how appetizing the dish itself looked; and (e) how much the resident enjoyed eating (Buckinx et al., 2017). While Buckinx and colleagues noted limited effect of the environment on residents' dining experiences, what seemed to be most important was resident perception; as residents' positive perceptions increased, so did their satisfaction with the meal, service of food, and the quality of the experience itself, which was largely tied the quantity of food served. Other sample questions to assess resident dining satisfaction are included in Exhibit 6.5.

Exhibit 6.5 Sample Questions to Include on Resident Meal Satisfaction Surveys in Care Communities

- Rate the overall quality of meals with respect to:

  - Taste.
  - Appeal.
  - Texture.
  - Presentation.
  - Desirable foods.
  - Undesirable foods.

- Rate if the hot food is hot.
- Rate if the cold food is cold.
- Rate the appropriateness of portion sizes for meals served at the care community.
- Rate the dining atmosphere.
- Rate the variety of foods offered to residents.
- Rate the choices of food available to residents.
- Give an overall impression of the food service in the care community.
- Note the things that are good which should be continued.
- Note the things which could be improved relative to food service.

Adapted from "Culture Change: Improving Quality of Life by Enhancing Dining Experience in a Skilled Nursing Facility" (Bhat et al., 2016).

For residents with dementia or those that suffer from visual impairments, the use of contrasting, bright colors has been documented as important to aid in improving the meal experience and increasing the amount of food ingested by residents. While many facilities have opted to use plastic cups and silverware for residents with impairments, the implementation of traditional plates and metal silverware to re-create a more homelike meal experience can improve residents' experiences and food and fluid intake. Other facilities have transformed their dining experiences through hiring culinary-trained chefs and waitstaff in crisp uniforms to promote a restaurant dining experience, complete with table linens, water goblets, and menus with multiple offerings. Even the eating process itself can be made easier and more pleasurable if dishes in contrasting colors to table coverings and food are used, as it is more difficult for a resident to navigate the food landscape if mashed potatoes are served on a white plate which is placed on an ivory tablecloth, and spills are more likely if black coffee is served in a dark-colored mug (Fig. 6.6).

One personal item that also plays into the ambiance of the dining experience is the potential use of clothing protectors, which should really be the autonomous choice of each individual resident. Some residents may see them as undignified and do not want to be forced to wear a "bib," while others see food spills on clothing as a dignity issue and would much prefer using a clothing protector during meals to prevent them. There are many modern clothing protectors that serve as a barrier to protect from food spills that no longer look like traditional bibs—including styles that simply look like large napkins, with closures for easy on-off use, or even protectors designed to look like shirt fronts, so when forward-facing, individuals appear to be wearing a regular shirt.

Beyond the table and flatware, the ambiance in the dining room has the opportunity to positively affect residents. Many care centers have employed quiet music during meal times as it has been shown to decrease resident agitation (Aldridge, 2007; Hicks-Moore, 2005), especially for residents with dementia, such as Alzheimer's disease (Thomas & Smith, 2009). Such use of relaxing music choices "buffers the general noise level typically found in dining rooms of nursing homes"

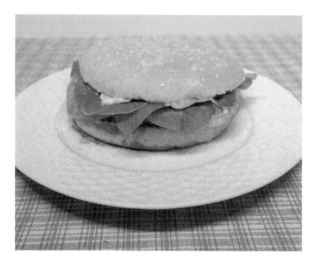

Fig. 6.6 Food which contrasts in color with the plate it is served on, which in turn contrasts with the tablecloth, placemat, or color of the table itself, aids residents with dementia or those residents who have visual impairments at meal times. Vividly distinguishable colors both improves the amount of food consumed by residents and can also be done in a manner that creates a more homelike environment for residents during meals. Photo Credit: Alena Shekhovtcova

(Aldridge, 2007) and can result in increased caloric intake and more time spent by residents in the dining environment (Thomas & Smith, 2009). Important also is the choice of music, where effective utilization during dining experiences includes music that residents prefer or that evokes pleasant memories from former stages of life. In some cases, studies have noted that the presence of music can increase agitation and distraction during mealtimes, having a deleterious effect on food consumption, so thoughtful use and appropriately crafted playlists based on resident preferences do matter.

6.6   Essential Influencers

A myriad of personnel, inside and outside the dietary department, play important roles in ensuring residents have high-quality, enjoyable dining experiences in care centers.

6.6.1   Dieticians and Dietary Managers

Primarily involved in the selection of resident meals in long-term care settings, to ensure appropriate nutrition and hydration, is the dietician or certified dietary manager. Some facilities also use the terms Director of Food Service, Culinary Director, or similar titles for these positions. In US care communities, this role can be supported by a "dietetic technician, registered" (DTR), a person who is trained and educated to provide meals and hydration that ensure healthy, culturally sensitive, quality food for residents and who works under the supervision of a registered dietitian nutritionist (RDN). In coordinating the food selection, some care communities have formed resident advisory committees to aid Food Service Directors, RDNs, and DTRs in crafting menus that will excite and satiate residents' appetites, and other facilities have turned to the existing resident council in the building to get feedback on what to add, remove, or revamp to cater to residents' preferences.

6.6.2   Medical Director and Therapists

For residents who require a modified diet or substituted items due to physical or cognitive impairment (e.g., residents rehabilitating following a stroke, residents with dysphagia, residents with Alzheimer's disease), the involvement of the facility medical director and therapists (e.g., speech-language pathologists, occupational therapists) may be required. Appropriate care plans should be developed to utilize nutritional foods and appropriate hydration, even when substitutions are required, that are palatable, presented in a similar style as non-modified food would be, and are in accordance with resident preferences, whenever possible. The medical director and therapists are essential personnel to consult, in addition to the resident, to ensure residents enjoy meal times even when modified for any impaired abilities. Additionally, the use of adaptive equipment or specialized flatware or drinkware may be an essential area where therapists and the medical director could be consulted.

6.6.3   Dietary Aides

When food is delivered to residents, many care centers employ dietary aides to assist in this process. Such aides also may assist residents during meal times if there are physical or cognitive impairments that may inhibit the resident from feeding himself or herself independently. In many care centers, to infuse elements of hospitality and progress away from the medical model of care delivery, dietary aides have been re-named as "servers" or "waiters" to more closely imitate restaurant-style dining, and some buildings use the term "nutrition assistants" for these staff members, too. Much as a server might respond to customers in a restaurant, dietary aides, too, can be trained (and often naturally evolve) to anticipate resident needs and respond timely to further improve the dining experience.

For many care communities, food is prepared in one location (e.g., larger kitchen areas) by cooks or chefs, and then delivered to residents in smaller dining areas throughout the building. To more fully embrace notions of culture change, some care communities have also placed a "chef" out at a cooking station in the smaller dining area to concoct a delicious meal, such as an omelet station for breakfast that allows residents to select their desired ingredients and then have the chef combine and prepare their meal in front of them. If food is served using a tray to assist staff members, plates and dishes should be removed from the tray and placed in front of the resident, to create and maintain a homelike dining experience.

6.6.4   Nurse Aides

In response to staffing shortages in many care communities, administrators and executive directors have implemented cross-training strategies, where one staff member is trained to do a multitude of tasks within a building. This strategy is often employed in smaller long-term care settings, such as the Green House homes, where one staff member performs several functions to assist residents. Under this approach, nurse aides (i.e., CNAs, PCAs) and housekeeping staff may also assist during meal times, especially if they have the ability to cook alongside the resident and prepare a meal together, which can occur in smaller care settings and with residents who enjoy cooking. This shared experience has the very real potential to strengthen the bond between caregivers and residents and can enhance the meal itself, as aides often are the staff who know the most about residents and are often the most informed to help ensure appropriate meal choices are available, including snacks and beverages throughout the day.

References

Aldridge, D. (2007). Dining rituals and music. *Music Therapy Today, 8*(1), 26–38.

Amarantos, E., Martinez, A., & Dwyer, J. (2001). Nutrition and quality of life in older adults. *Journals of Gerontology, Series A: Biological Sciences and Medical Sciences, 56*(Suppl_2), 54–64. https://doi.org/10.1093/gerona/56.suppl_2.54

American Medical Directors Association. (2010). *Altered nutritional status in the long-term care setting: Clinical practice guideline.* Retrieved from: https://paltc.org/topic/nutrition (August 2021).

Bhat, C. J., Wagle, A., McProud, L., & Ousey, S. (2016). Culture change: Improving quality of life by enhancing dining experience in a skilled nursing facility. *Journal of Foodservice Business Research, 19*(3), 287–297. https://doi.org/10.1080/15378020.2016.1175901

Bowman, C. S. (2010, June). *The food and dining side of the culture change movement: Identifying barriers and potential solutions to furthering innovation in nursing homes.* Pre-Symposium Paper. Presented at the Creating Home in the Nursing Home II: A National Symposium on Culture Change and the Food and Dining Requirements. Retrieved from: https://www.pioneernetwork.net/wp-content/uploads/2016/10/The-Food-and-Dining-Side-of-the-Culture-Change-Movement-Symposium-Background-Paper.pdf.

Buckinx, F., Reginster, J., Morelle, A., Paquot, N., Labeye, N., Locquet, M., Adam, S., & Bruyère, O. (2017). Influence of environmental factors on food intake among nursing home residents: A survey combined with a video approach. *Clinical Interventions in Aging, 12*, 1055–1064.

Centers for Medicare and Medicaid Services, United States Department of Health and Human Services. (2009). *Nursing home requirements for food procurement, self determination, and participation.* Retrieved from: https://www.cms.gov/Medicare/Provider-Enrollment-and-Certification/SurveyCertificationGenInfo/Policy-and-Memos-to-States-and-Regions-Items/CMS1222974.

Desai, J., Winter, A., Young, K. W. H., & Greenwood, C. E. (2007). Changes in type of foodservice and dining room environment preferentially benefit institutionalized seniors with low body mass indexes. *Journal of the American Dietetic Association, 107*, 808–814.

Divert, C., Laghmaoui, R., Crema, C., Issanchou, S., Van Wymelbeke, V., & Sulmont-Rossé, C. (2015). Improving meal context in nursing homes. Impact of four strategies on food intake and meal pleasure. *Appetite, 84*, 139–147.

Dunn, H., & Moore, T. (2016). "You can't be forcing food down 'em": Nursing home carers' perceptions of residents' dining needs. *Journal of Health Psychology, 21*(5), 619–627. https://doi.org/10.1177/1359105314532971

Engh, M. C. N., & Speyer, R. (2020). Management of dysphagia in nursing homes: A national survey. *Dysphagia, 37*(2), 266–276. https://doi.org/10.1007/s00455-021-10275-7

Green House Project. (2021, July). *Revolutionizing care to empower lives.* Retrieved from: https://thegreenhouseproject.org/our-story/who-we-are/.

Harper, C., Cullen, P., & Fodey, K. (2014). *Nutritional guidelines and menu checklist for residential and nursing homes.* Retrieved from: http://www.efad.org/media/1351/nutritional_guidlines_and_menu_checklist_march_2014.pdf.

Hicks-Moore, S. L. (2005). Relaxing music at mealtime in nursing homes: Effects on agitated patients with dementia. *Journal of Gerontological Nursing, 31*(12), 26–32.

Hotaling, D. L. (1990). Adapting the mealtime environment: Setting the state for eating. *Dysphagia, 5*, 77–83.

Johnstone, A. (2018). *How your age affects your appetite*. BBC 100 year life series. Retrieved from: https://www.bbc.com/future/article/20180629-the-seven-stages-of-life-that-affect-how-we-eat.

Kane, R. L., Rockwood, T., Hyer, K., Desjardins, K., Brassard, A., Gessert, C., & Kane, R. (2005). Rating the importance of nursing home residents' quality of life. *Journal of the American Geriatrics Society, 53*, 2076–2082.

Kuosma, K., Hjerrild, J., Pedersen, P. U., & Hundrup, Y. A. (2008). Assessment of the nutritional status among residents in a Danish nursing home: Health effects of a formulated food and meal policy. *Journal of Clinical Nursing, 17*, 2288–2293. https://doi.org/10.1111/j.1365-2702.2007.02203.x

Lowndes, R., Armstrong, P., & Daly, T. (2015). The meaning of "dining": The social organization of food in long-term care. *Food Studies, 4*(1), 19–34.

MacIntosh, W. A., Shifflett, P. A., & Picou, P. J. (1989). Social support, stressful events, strain, dietary intake and the elderly. *Medical Care, 27*(2), 140–153.

McColl, S. (2015, July). *Farm-to-table dining hits the retirement home*. TakePart. Retrieved from: http://www.takepart.com/article/2015/08/12/elder-care-farm-table.

Milwaukee Catholic Home (2020, June). *Clare gardens*. Retrieved from: https://www.milwaukeecatholichome.org/community-life/claregardens/.

Nijs, K., de Graaf, C., Blauw, Y., Vanneste, V., Kok, F., & van Staveren, W. (2006). Effect of family-style meals on energy intake and risk of malnutrition in Dutch nursing home residents: A randomized controlled trial. *The Journals of Gerontology: Series A, 61*(9), 935–942. https://doi.org/10.1093/gerona/61.9.935

O'Loughlin, G., & Shanley, C. (1998). Swallowing problems in the nursing home: A novel training response. *Dysphagia, 13*, 172–183.

Robinson, G. E., & Gallagher, A. (2008). Culture change impacts quality of life for nursing home residents. *Topics in Clinical Nutrition, 23*(2), 120–130.

Simmons, S. F., Keeler, E., Zhuo, X., Hickey, K. A., Sato, H., & Schnelle, J. F. (2008). Prevention of unintentional weight loss in nursing home residents: A controlled trial of feeding assistance. *Journal of the American Geriatrics Society, 56*, 1466–1473.

Skilled Nursing News. (2021, July). *Skilled nursing dining in 2021: Industry survey report*. Retrieved from: https://skillednursingnews.com.

Speroff, B. A., Davis, K. H., & Dehr, K. L. (2005). The dining experience in nursing homes. *North Carolina Medical Journal, 66*(4), 292–295.

Stange, I., Bartram, M., Liao, Y., Poeschl, K., Kolpatzik, S., Uter, W., Sieber, C. C., Stehle, P., & Volkert, D. (2013). Effects of a low-volume, nutrient- and energy-dense oral nutritional supplement on nutritional and functional status: A randomized, controlled trial in nursing home residents. *Journal of the American Medical Directors Association, 14*(8), 628.e1–628.e8. https://doi.org/10.1016/j.jamda.2013.05.011

Stange, I., Poeschl, K., Stehle, P., Sieber, C. C., & Volkert, D. (2013). Screening for malnutrition in nursing home residents: Comparison of different risk markers and their association to functional impairment. *Journal of Nutrition, Health, and Aging, 17*, 357–363. https://doi.org/10.1007/s12603-013-0021-z

Steele, C. M., Namasivayam-MacDonald, A. M., Guida, B. T., Hanson, B., Lam, P., & Riquelme, L. F. (2018). Creation and initial validation of the international dysphagia diet standardisation initiative functional diet scale. *Archives of Physical Medicine and Rehabilitation, 99*(5), 934–944. https://doi.org/10.1016/j.apmr.2018.01.012

Thomas, D. W., & Smith, M. (2009). The effect of music on caloric consumption among nursing home residents with dementia of the Alzheimer's type. *Activities, Adaptation and Aging, 33*(1), 1–16. https://doi.org/10.1080/01924780902718566

Van Wymelbeke, V., Sulmont-Rossé, C., Feyen, V., Issanchou, S., Manckoundia, P., & Maître, I. (2020). Optimizing sensory quality and variety: An effective strategy for increasing meal enjoyment and food intake in older nursing home residents. *Appetite, 153*, 104749.

Verbrugghe, M., Beeckman, D., Van Hecke, A., Vanderwee, K., Van Herck, K., Clays, E., Bocquaert, I., Derycke, H., Geurden, B., & Verhaeghe, S. (2013). Malnutrition and associated factors in nursing home residents: A cross-sectional, multi-Centre study. *Clinical Nutrition, 32*(3), 438–443. https://doi.org/10.1016/j.clnu.2012.09.008

Watson, R. (1993). Measuring feeding difficulty in patients with dementia: Perspectives and problems. *Journal of Advanced Nursing, 18*, 25–31.

Young, K. W., Binns, M. A., & Greenwood, C. E. (2001). Meal delivery practices do not meet needs of Alzheimer patients with increased cognitive and behavioral difficulties in a long-term care facility. *Journals of Gerontology, Series A: Biological Sciences and Medical Sciences, 56*, M656–M661.

Chapter 7
Quality of Care

We've been wrong about what our job is in medicine. We think our job is to ensure health and survival. But really it is larger than that. It is to enable well-being. – Atul Gawande

Abstract In this penultimate chapter, the medical aspects of care provided in long-term care settings are emphasized. Some of the existing literature distinguishes quality of care from quality of life, while other research explores the interrelated nature of the two concepts. This relationship is explored in depth, emphasizing the importance of individualized medical care (e.g., nursing care and services, specialty care, physical therapy, occupational therapy) aspects provided to residents and how care can impact quality of life, including the Centers for Medicare and Medicaid Services-enumerated quality measures for short-stay and long-stay residents. While somewhat related, the chapter also includes a brief discussion of the problem of elder maltreatment within care communities across the globe. The care planning processes and incorporation of residents, residents' family members, or residents' proxy decision-makers in the process are emphasized, as are the inclusion of unique resident-driven preferences and needs to tailor care plans appropriately. Finally, the importance of transitions (i.e., transfers) between various care settings is addressed (e.g., hospital discharge to nursing home for therapy), as poorly executed transfers have negative implications on resident health and quality of life (e.g., transfer trauma, increased cognitive decline, disorientation).

Keywords Quality of care · Medical care · Quality measures · Quality of life · Nursing · Specialized units · Nursing home · Assisted living center · Physical therapy · Occupational therapy · Speech-language pathology · Care planning · Care plans · Discharge · Re-hospitalization · Proxy decision-makers · Resident-centered care · Resident-directed care · Transfers of care · Role of staff

The care needs of older adults continue to become more complex (Castle, 2008), with contemporary nursing homes often focusing on two primary types of residents: short-stay residents, recuperating post-surgery or post-hospitalization, and long-stay residents, who come to a care community with physical or cognitive impairments and will live there for the remainder of their days. For those residents in an assisted living center, medical care onsite may be less essential, as these residents often have higher physical and cognitive functioning (even though some assisted living centers provide basic memory care), hence their ability to live in such a setting rather than one with greater amounts of medical care provided to residents with more complicated health conditions. Residents in care communities are often more vulnerable to lapses in appropriate care, due to their acuity level, because of deteriorations in physical and cognitive health, making the quality of their care an important consideration for administrators and staff members. Exhibit 7.1 displays common deficiencies assessed against nursing homes in the United States for poor quality of care. While there is an emphasis on managing or preventing additional chronic conditions, residents in care centers experience higher levels of morbidity and impairment, by definition, than their community-dwelling peers (Davis, 1991). It has become increasingly important over time to assess and ensure the quality of care provided to residents with physical and cognitive impairments.

Exhibit 7.1 Most Frequently Issued Deficiency Citations in United States Nursing Homes
- Food storage, preparation, and serving meals to residents.
- Accidents, hazards for residents, and improper supervision.
- Infection control programs.
- Quality of care.
- Appropriate background checks for nursing home staff members.
- Appropriate standards of quality in care center.
- Comprehensive care plans for residents.
- Residents not given unnecessary drugs.
- Appropriate policies and practices to prevent maltreatment.
- Housekeeping and maintenance.
- Maintenance of residents' records.
- Urinary incontinence.
- Pressure sores or pressure ulcers.
- Qualified staff members providing care and services in care centers.

Adapted from "Analyses of Complaints, Investigation of Allegations, and Deficiency Citations in United States Nursing Homes" (Hansen et al., 2019).

Quality of care has primarily been viewed as the medical aspect of care delivery within residential care settings, while quality of life has often been conceptualized in terms of resident satisfaction with the quality of care received and their perceptions of care center's environment. However, some researchers have contemplated these two aspects separately and distinct from one another, while other analyses argue the inherent interaction between the care provided and its impact on residents' satisfaction and quality of life. Recent evidence suggests, though, that residents receiving a higher quality of care don't always think about the impact of care quality, but when the quality of care is poor, it can and does substantially, negatively impact quality of life for care recipients (Johs-Artisensi et al., 2020).

7.1 Quality of Care

Some studies have suggested that, on average, for-profit nursing homes have poorer quality of care than their nonprofit counterparts, and nonprofit nursing homes have often been found to be more resident-centered and tend to prioritize "medical and personal aspects of care," which has been theorized to promote higher quality for residents (e.g., Amirkhanyan et al., 2008) (Fig. 7.1). Quality of care in US nursing homes is often analyzed using the proxy measure of deficiency citations a care center receives on its annual regulatory survey, both in quantity and severity of the deficiencies (Arling et al. 2007; Castle, 2002, 2011; Hansen et al., 2019; Harrington et al., 2004). A citation is issued when the provider is operating out of compliance with regulations that set minimum standards for care and operations. Upon receiving a citation, a nursing home is required to develop a plan of correction to remedy the noted deficiency (Castle, 2011), in efforts to bring the care center back into compliance with standards designed to assure appropriate quality of care and quality of life. Beyond deficiency citations, adverse resident outcomes such as death rates, potential re-hospitalizations, and nursing home discharges are often variables of interest when analyzing nursing home quality (Anderson et al., 1998). In the United States, another proxy measure utilized to gauge quality of care are resident-specific quality measures. These measures have been distinguished for the short-stay resident receiving rehabilitative therapy services separate from the quality measures designed for long-stay residents, where the care center is now their new home, and include such metrics as the percent of residents receiving antipsychotic medications, percent of residents with a pressure ulcer (pressure sore), or percent of residents with high self-reported pain.

When budgets are tight, care communities may attempt to reduce expenditures on resident care, often in the form of lower quality staffing, which has the potential to increase the rate of adverse events (Comondore et al., 2009). Some research has indicated that persistently poor-quality nursing homes tended to maintain a poor level of quality over a period of time, whereas higher-quality nursing homes tended to maintain a higher level of quality during the same period (Grabowski & Castle, 2004; Mor et al., 2004). Care centers in states that provided overall better reimbursement for care (i.e., reimbursement covered more of the actual expenses of providing care to residents) tended to start and remain as high-quality facilities (Grabowski & Castle, 2004). When resources are limited and, thusly, facilities reduce care or services provided, this has the very real potential to diminish resident quality of care and, eventually, quality of life (Fig. 7.2).

Care communities that employ a greater percentage of registered nurses (RNs) and certified nursing assistants (CNAs) among on-duty staff tend to deliver better

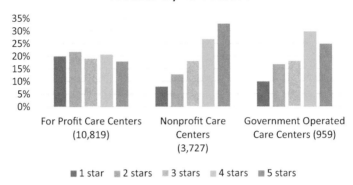

Star Ratings for United States Nursing Homes by Tax Status

Fig. 7.1 For profit nursing homes in the United States have been shown to have overall lower quality than their nonprofit counterparts, and there are many more for profit facilities than there are nonprofit sites. Adapted from the Kaiser Family Foundation's "Reading the Stars: Nursing Home Quality Star Ratings, Nationally and by State" (2015)

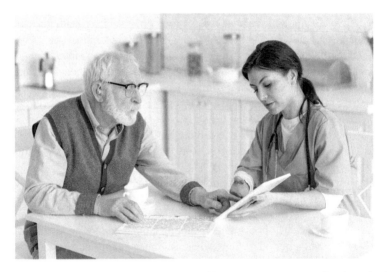

Fig. 7.2 Nursing staff in care centers are an invaluable resource to assure continual monitoring of resident health and medical needs. While sheer numbers of nursing staff (including RNs, licensed practical nurses [LPN/LVNs], and CNAs) are important to consider, *how* the staff members utilize their expertise in the care setting is almost as important, too. Some care centers have moved toward cross-training their CNA staff members to have a greater ability to consistently work with a smaller subset of residents and work to better tailor care to those individuals. Photo Credit: U.S. Veterans Health Administration

quality of care (Anderson et al., 1998). However, the structure, staff skill mix, and delivery of care according to evidence-based practices may even more directly affect quality of care than merely having enough staff members on duty (Arling et al. 2007a; Castle & Ferguson, 2010; Davis, 1991). Others have analyzed the relationship between staffing and quality of care measures, finding that higher staffing levels often indicated higher quality (Castle, 2008) (see Exhibit 7.2). An increased number of direct care staff (e.g., CNAs) has been shown to be significantly related to better restorative care (e.g., activities of daily living [ADL] training), which enhances the quality of care given within a particular facility (Arling et al., 2007a). Facilities with lower staffing levels (e.g., RNs, CNAs) have been shown to use practices that can diminish a resident's quality of life, such as the use of restraints, especially when residents are dependent upon staff for ADL assistance (Arling et al., 2007a). CNA staffing levels, as well as how CNAs are utilized within a particular care center (e.g., cross-trained staff to help with various services) can also predict lower total deficiency scores and lower quality of care deficiency scores within nursing homes (Hyer et al., 2011), thus leading to better care for residents.

Exhibit 7.2 The Relationship Between Nurse Staffing Levels and Quality of Care

- Higher staffing levels of CNAs in a care center resulted in lower numbers of deficiency citations overall and lower numbers of citations related to quality of care issues.
- For every increase of CNA hours in a care center, there is a corresponding reduction in deficient quality care (conversely, nursing homes with one hour fewer of CNAs per resident day have an increase in the number of quality of care citations issued to them).
- The recommended staffing level for CNAs is 4.1 total hours per resident day, per the United States Centers for Medicare and Medicaid Services.
- Licensed nursing (e.g., RNs, LPN/LVNs) was found to not be significantly related to deficiency scores when factoring in CNA nursing hours.

Adapted from "The Influence of Nurse Staffing Levels on Quality of Care in Nursing Homes" (Hyer et al., 2011).

7.2 Intersection of Care and Quality of Life

Nursing home quality of life has been characterized as distinct from the clinical care received by residents, even in studies attempting to document a relationship between quality of care and quality of life (Degenholtz et al., 2006). Donabedian (1988) argued for further analyses into the interaction between residents and staff members to determine how such interactions affect resident health and welfare, which is covered in more detail in the Relationships with Other Residents, Staff, and Family Members chapter. It has also been suggested that quality of life indicators (e.g.,

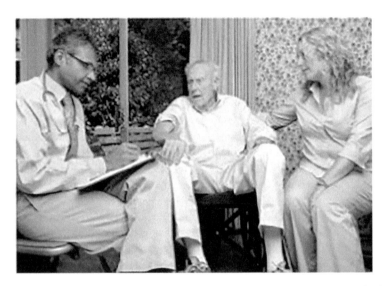

Fig. 7.3 The facility's medical director—one of the key members on the care center leadership team—has a key role to play in providing the highest possible quality of care to residents in the building. Given the dearth of geriatrics residencies in many medical schools, the vast majority of long-term care medical directors have come from other areas of practice (e.g., general practice physician, pediatrician) and adapt their experience to an older adult population. As residents' health conditions change over time, a proactive medical director will work with nursing staff and other specialists, as needed, to adapt the care plan and respond appropriately to what the resident may need. Photo Credit: Hay Dmitriy

functional ability, behaviors related to dementia, usage of restraints) have the ability to predict resident outcomes better than some quality of care measures (e.g., pressure sores, indwelling catheters, urinary tract infections) as they "directly relate to residents' conditions" (Anderson et al., 1998) (Fig. 7.3).

Relationships appear to exist between residents' self-reported quality of life and clinical quality of care metrics (e.g., quality measures, physical and psychosocial well-being) taken from standardized assessments of care center residents (Degenholtz et al., 2006). Exhibit 7.3 displays questions that care centers can use to assess resident satisfaction levels with the quality of care provided. Changes in the quality of care provided to residents can affect quality of life, even when adjusting for resident-specific factors. There have been within-facility variations noted relative to quality of life that residents experience as influenced by varying quality of care approaches and whether care is individualized and tailored to residents appropriately. The quality of care measures noted above have been demonstrated to affect overall quality of life, and while sometimes quality of care indicators have also been used to measure quality of life, the latter is less common.

Exhibit 7.3 Sample Customer Satisfaction Survey Questions Related to Quality of Care (for Residents with and Without Dementia)

Where possible, the following questions should be asked directly to residents, whether in person or through an anonymous form for the resident to complete, to promote candid responses with anonymity. If a resident has cognitive impairment to the degree they cannot respond, then proxy individuals (e.g., spouse, family members) should be used to complete the survey questionnaire.

- I feel the CNAs like their job.
- I feel the RNs and LPN/LVNs like their job.
- The nursing staff understand how residents feel and what their preferences are.
- The nurses and staff are well trained.
- The staff cares about residents.
- Adequate therapy time is available for my needs.
- Numerous changes in staff members upsets my routine.
- The administrator (or executive director) considers suggestions from residents and family for changing care practices in the care center.
- If requested, residents will get a change in their care practices or staff members providing care.
- The dietician is easy to talk with.
- The therapists (e.g., physical therapist, occupational therapist, speech-language therapist) are easy to talk with and respect my preferences during therapy sessions.
- The medical director is easy to talk with and respects my preferences when engaging in care planning.
- The staff members deal honestly with residents in their interactions.

Adapted from "The Silent Customers: Measuring Customer Satisfaction in Nursing Homes" (Kleinsorge & Koenig, 1991) and "Definition, Measurement, and Correlates of Quality of Life in Nursing Homes: Toward a Reasonable Practice, Research, and Policy Agenda" (R. A. Kane, 2003).

Individual resident characteristics and resident self-assessments of quality have been shown to be better predictors of quality of life, as compared to aggregate facility characteristics based on all residents in a particular building. This is especially true when residents maintained some cognitive, functional abilities and had an engaging social environment (Shippee et al., 2013). Although resident satisfaction alone is often used as a measure of quality of life, various researchers have attempted to develop more comprehensive tools to measure this important, but elusive, concept. A six-item instrument was developed that includes measuring satisfaction with RNs and CNAs, administration, empathy (or concern) for residents, food quality, housekeeping quality, and issues within the nursing home (Kleinsorge & Koenig, 1991). R. A. Kane (2003) posits that analyses of quality of life must include the resident's "voice" in ascertaining operational definitions for quality of life in care centers, and enumerates five necessary steps for designing a quality of life measurement tool: (a) designing appropriate questions, (b) creating a sampling strategy, (c) collecting necessary resident-level and facility-level variables, (d) validating constructs used, and (e) developing proxy measures for residents too impaired to contribute. Further studies in quality of life have found that facility-level factors (e.g., profit status, private vs. non-private or semi-private rooms, location) provide an opportunity to distinguish high-quality facilities from low-quality facilities based on resident self-reported quality of life (R. L. Kane et al., 2004).

Somewhere at the intersection of care and quality of life lies a problematic issue that can negatively affect care communities—namely, elder maltreatment. Research into the problem of abuse and neglect in facility-based settings continues to evolve and better address the complexities of these forms of maltreatment (Lindbloom et al., 2007), though comprehensive data on the prevalence of maltreatment in long-term care settings is lacking (Teaster et al., 2007). Incidents of resident abuse in nursing homes affect quality of life beyond just concerns for resident health and safety (Castle, 2011; Jogerst et al., 2006). Approximately 79% of staff members in German nursing homes indicated, in self-report questionnaires, they had abused (verbal abuse, in most instances) or neglected a resident and 66% observed maltreatment of residents by a co-worker but did nothing (Goergen, 2001). In Australia, residents who suffered an incident of abuse had subsequent increased levels of disability, and abuse incidents that involved coercion and feelings of dejection post-victimization were associated with higher rates of mortality (Schofield et al., 2013). If abuse and neglect occur, one cannot argue that an optimal or high quality of care was provided to the resident, and such maltreatment has obvious implications on substantially reducing a resident's quality of life and feelings of safety in their home.

7.3 Measuring and Assuring Quality

Although there is no single resident outcome measure that sufficiently captures quality of care, quality of life, nor resource allocation, clearly, quality of care can have a significant impact on resident quality of life. Quality of care is affected by many stakeholders: residents, their families, staff and administration, the medical director, the director of nursing (DON), policy makers, and more (Davis, 1991). Resident quality of care is a multifaceted concept and is affected by numerous factors present within a nursing home environment (e.g., staffing levels, training for staff, condition of equipment or medical devices, availability of necessary resources to provide care). By definition, long-term care occurs over a significant period of time, so it is important to routinely monitor and assess care delivery practices on a regular basis to constantly improve residents' experiences.

Prior to admission, residents and their families often do not have sufficient information to make an informed choice on which care center to select based on its quality of care provided to residents (Spector et al., 1998). This is true for nursing homes, and even more so the case for assisted living facilities where there are very few reported public metrics in many cases. Certain initiatives have been pursued to remedy the lack of information, such as the Care Compare website in the United States, maintained by the Centers for Medicare and Medicaid Services (CMS), which compares a nursing home against state and national averages for various scores on the quality of care provided (see Exhibit 7.4). These scores are largely based upon the nursing home quality measures that analyze facility performance in care delivery and resident outcomes (Arling et al., 2007b) for both short-stay and long-stay residents. Examples of these nursing home quality measures include the percentage of residents with a urinary tract infection, residents who were physically restrained, residents who received an antipsychotic medication, residents who are high-risk that have pressure ulcers, and more (CMS, 2020). Assisted living facilities are not included in Care Compare, however, and there is no comparable equivalent to aid consumers in selecting a new residence, other than private companies that charge facilities to be listed on their site or consumer-driven reviews posted to Google or social media sites (e.g., Facebook).

Exhibit 7.4 Metrics of Quality to Evaluate Care Centers in the United States

- Overall star rating (out of five stars total) for the care center, comprised of several of the following metrics.
- Health inspections star rating, on CMS Care Compare, and deficiencies given to each care center on an approximately-annual basis.
- Number of complaints levied against the care center, as well as the number and date of investigations into allegations raised.
- Number of infection control inspections at each care center, as well as any citations issued for poor quality.
- Staffing level star rating, which are reported electronically each quarter by care centers and verified by surveyors during annual inspections.
- Quality of resident care star rating, measured through defined, separate medical care metrics for short-stay and long-stay residents in the care center.
- All fines and fees paid by the care center within the preceding three years (e.g., penalties for poor quality related to care and services for residents).
- Demographics of the care center, including profit status (e.g., for profit vs. nonprofit entity), whether the care center has a resident or family council (or both), and the payer sources accepted at the care center (e.g., Medicare, Medicaid).

Metrics included are publicly available on the federal Care Compare website, with data maintained and updated annually by the Centers for Medicare and Medicaid Services, United States Department of Health and Human Services (2021).

When analyzing quality of care to improve processes affecting residents, there are often three main factors examined: (a) care provided by specific care center staff members; (b) care received by residents (e.g., short-stay or long-stay residents, or both); and (c) the capacity of providers to deliver the care to residents (Donabedian, 2005). Some of the primary quality indicators used for analyses of facility-level quality include the size of the nursing home, financial costs for daily operations, staffing and staff composition, profit status (i.e., for-profit or nonprofit), and reimbursement methodologies for care delivered (e.g., private pay, governmental sources, private insurance) (Davis, 1991).

7.4 Providing Quality Resident Care and Therapy Services

The medical care provided to residents in care settings can vary greatly. To even be admitted to a care center, in some countries, prospective residents must demonstrate the need for assistance with multiple ADLs, such as dressing, eating, ambulating, toileting, bathing, and transferring. Beyond ADL assistance, many residents need additional medical care, including residents with cognitive impairment (e.g., dementia, Alzheimer's disease, Parkinson's disease, traumatic brain injuries), residents requiring bariatric care (i.e., for obesity), residents needing mechanical ventilation due to respiratory conditions, and other complex medical care. As noted above, modern-day nursing homes have also focused on rehabilitative care and specialized services for a number of acute conditions—for example, joint replacement, cardiac incidents, and strokes. Care centers sometimes serve as an essential transition between an acute care setting (e.g., hospitals) and the person's own home, providing physical therapy, occupational therapy, and speech-language therapy for rehabilitation (Fig. 7.4).

Residents in nursing homes have become more physically and cognitively impaired over time as more options have evolved for housing and services suitable for those with a lower acuity. In the United States, the advent of assisted living centers and senior living apartments (i.e., age-restricted buildings or organized housing) has meant that older adults who need minor assistance can instead elect to live in such settings and receive some limited assistance with daily needs. Assisted living centers, in many locations, provide a moderate level of care to residents with a lower acuity than would be in nursing homes (e.g., assistance with ADLs, medication distribution and reminders, memory care for residents with dementia, transferring residents with mobility issues). Other assisted living centers provide an even lower level of medical care and focus instead more on "hospitality" elements (e.g., provision of meals, social activities with other residents, emergency assistance when needed). Where once there was a standalone nursing home, now there are more and more settings that provide multiple lines of service so individuals can age in place through the continuum of long-term care (e.g., continuing care retirement centers).

As the physical impairment of residents has increased, as well as the growth in short-stay residents completing rehabilitation after a hospitalization or surgery, there

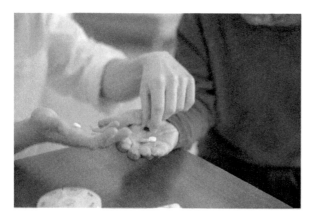

Fig. 7.4 Medication administration—or assistance taking required prescriptions—is an essential service offered to care center residents across various settings. When residents miss prescription medications, there can be more pronounced effects on health. Also, the care of the medical director and nursing staff to assure no contraindicated medications are taken by the resident is important, given the multiple medications taken by the majority of care center residents. Photo Credit: Kampus Production

has been a mirrored increase in therapy services provided. Many care centers have invested significant resources into creating therapy spaces, including the purchase of specialized equipment, to assist physical therapists, occupational therapists, and speech-language pathologists in the work they do to improve residents' health and ability to return home successfully to the community. Some care communities have exercise rooms that residents can use at their leisure, separate from specialized therapy provided with licensed or certified individuals that is tailored to a resident's particular needs. There is also some crossover with therapy and activities, where some care centers have pools for water aerobics or bring in community members to do chair yoga with residents—where an activity planned for social engagement can also have a medicinal or therapeutic benefit to the residents who participate, when thoughtfully planned and carefully executed with modifications to adapt to residents' abilities (Fig. 7.5). The inclusion of therapeutic activities has the benefit of increasing resident functionality and independence which, through care recipients' own reports, contributes to a higher, more positive quality of life in care centers (Johs-Artisensi et al., 2020).

In conjunction with the evolution of the long-term care continuum, some nursing homes have opted to specialize in the care of certain residents. Some nursing homes are designed and staffed to only serve residents who are ventilator-dependent due to pulmonary diseases or conditions (e.g., Dove Healthcare Wissota Health and Regional Vent Center, 2021). Another specialty pursued by some nursing homes is in the treatment of certain illnesses, such as one care community that exists primarily to serve residents with Huntington's Disease (e.g., Good Samaritan Society – Specialty Care Community, 2021). As the obesity rates have increased over time, some nursing homes also have specialized in care for obese individuals

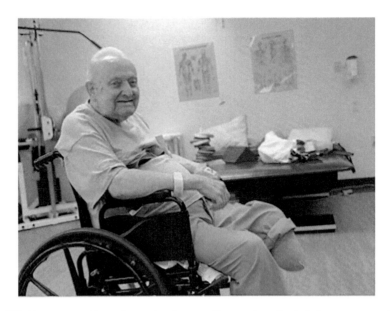

Fig. 7.5 Short-stay residents in nursing homes often receive physical therapy, occupational therapy, speech-language therapy, or some combination of these. Most care centers are equipped with therapy spaces that have traditional physical therapy equipment; washers, dryers, and other household items for occupational therapy; and separate spaces, in some facilities, where activities may be held with a physical exercise component (e.g., tai-chi or yoga in a large community center, water aerobics in a pool). Photo Credit: Marion Veterans Administration Medical Center

who require bariatric care and specialized equipment such as portable or ceiling lifts, reinforced wheelchairs, and modified bathing furniture and chairs (e.g., Wayne County Nursing Home and Rehab Center, 2021). For those care centers not specializing exclusively in one type of resident care, many have created specialized units or wings within a care center to provide specialized care for various unique populations. In providing services to distinct target populations, care centers can capitalize on the opportunity to further train staff members with specific education and skills designed to elevate the excellence of care provided to these residents.

Much like the specialized care communities noted above for select cognitive or physical impairments, so too have specialized facilities evolved to treat certain groups of individuals that may require more unique care. With the increase in life expectancy over time, certain groups of individuals that historically had higher mortality rates have been living longer, eventually requiring the level of medical care or services and supports provided within nursing homes and other long-term care settings. Such individuals include those residents with mental illness, behavioral disorders, intellectual (i.e., developmental) disabilities, and incarcerated persons. For example, a nursing home was built, licensed, and now operates to provide care and services to persons who are civilly committed (due to mental illness) or who have been incarcerated and require nursing home level of care (e.g., Forensic Nursing Home, Minnesota Department of Human Services, 2021). For adults with developmental disabilities, there are various forms of community-based living available (e.g., adult group homes), with the trend being that individuals with intellectual disabilities most often receive care and services outside of traditional long-term care settings (Landes & Lillaney, 2019). However, some individuals require more intensive care which might best be provided in a nursing home or other congregate care setting (e.g., Intermediate Care Facilities for Individuals with Intellectual Disabilities).

Beyond the care and services provided onsite in many care centers, residents may have other medical care needs that can be provided offsite by an independent provider or one with whom the facility has contracted to provide a service. This may include outpatient visits to primary or specialty care physicians, as well as dental care and optometry services, to name a few. Care centers are typically obligated to ensure residents can make and attend their appointments for offsite care, which may necessitate the arrangement of transportation services by family members, through a contracted non-emergency medical transportation service, or by a facility-operated vehicle that assists residents in getting to appointments.

7.5   Care Planning for Residents

Effective care planning (or care conferences) in care centers is inherently an inter-disciplinary process, and in many cases, also a required written document to ensure care is appropriately individualized and delivered to residents (Dellefield, 2006). When care plans are carefully crafted, they serve an important function to ensure care aligns with resident preferences, needs, wants, and cultural and religious beliefs, but also establish goals for resident care and expected timeframes to achieve certain outcomes.

Contemporary nomenclature often refers to much of the care and decision-making in nursing homes and assisted living centers as "resident-centered" or "person-centered." This is true as well for care planning processes. Incorporation of residents in the care planning process, dependent upon the resident's desire to be involved (e.g., some more introverted or reserved residents may not wish to have as active a role in the care planning that occurs), is an essential practice that care communities must employ. With the resident engaged as an active participant, directing the goals established in the plan and the inclusion of care that meets the resident's psychosocial, cultural, and spiritual needs—in addition to providing required medical care—care plans are more effective and can assist staff as they strive to provide a high quality of life in addition to care received. Often, residents may wish to include family members or proxy decision-makers (e.g., an agent appointed under a health care directive), which should be respected and honored. Especially for residents with cognitive impairments, family members, friends, or proxies may be able to "fill in the gaps" as far as what the resident may or may not enjoy, routines or patterns the resident may have had prior to residing at the care community, and share other helpful information to individualize care. In addition to

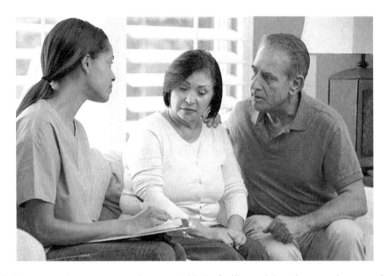

Fig. 7.6 Residents in care centers often meet with the facility social worker to update care plans as their health status changes over time. Care planning can be done in a resident-centered or person-centered way to ensure physical care needs are met, but also that resident preferences, wishes, and goals are met to heighten the quality of life in the care center. While residents should always be engaged in this process, some may prefer a spouse or family member participate to assist in articulating their wishes, including in cases where dementia may inhibit a resident's ability to do so. Photo Credit: US Bureau of Labor Statistics

involving proxies in care planning, facilities can also incorporate a resident's wishes that may have been stated in a properly created health care directive or advance directive (previously called a "power of attorney for health care"), which are created when the resident has capacity and articulates their health care wishes and care preferences in a document that can be shared with care providers in various care settings (Fig. 7.6).

Care planning often is built on standardized assessments of residents, typically conducted on initial admission to the care community and at regular, routine intervals thereafter to ensure any changes in resident functioning are appropriately incorporated into care and services provided. Such assessments often document a resident's physical and medical needs, but also incorporate preferences, cultural or spiritual beliefs and practices, and psychosocial needs. In addition to standardized assessments, other relevant information learned by nurses, CNAs, housekeepers, or dietary aides in their daily interactions with residents should be incorporated into care plans to best tailor care for each resident. Such input from staff members is helpful, even though care planning is generally conducted by the medical team in care centers (e.g., the medical director, DON, rehabilitation staff, social worker).

7.6   Transfers between Care Settings

One important aspect of the quality of care provided to residents is when a transition of care occurs between care settings or between a care setting and the resident's home. For short-term residents in care communities, transfers or transitions often occur following an acute care procedure (e.g., knee or hip replacement, cardiac procedure, treatment for a stroke) for rehabilitation and recuperation. As noted by Naylor & Keating (2008), "high-quality transitional care is especially important for older adults with multiple chronic conditions and complex therapeutic regimens," which is an apt descriptor of the typical nursing home resident. Besides relocating back home, transfers also may occur to another long-term care center. This may happen when a short-term resident has improved enough to step down to a lower level of care, such as an assisted living facility, or conversely, if care needs have heightened, the resident may need to move to a provider who offers care for more complex conditions. Additionally, long-term care is in a state of flux, and nursing home closures in the United States and Europe are not uncommon (Castle et al., 2009; Netten et al., 2003), necessitating a mass transfer or relocation of all their residents. In those cases, a thorough process, with the thoughtful inclusion of the resident and open communication by both the sending and receiving facilities, is critical to facilitating the adjustment process and achieving positive outcomes for residents and facilities (Johs-Artisensi, 2009).

A key component in a successful transfer is the sharing of medical records between care settings, which can go awry in many cases given the data systems used in specific care settings cannot always be shared with ease, even with resident consent, between care settings. In addition to sharing care information, proper communication between the discharge planner at the hospital and the admissions coordinator at the nursing home (both roles are usually filled by social workers) is also essential to ensure a successful "handoff" and continuity of care. Poor transitions have been shown to result in transfer trauma, increased cognitive decline for residents with dementia, enhanced disorientation of the resident, and, in some unfortunate cases, increased mortality.

When the resident is in the long-term care center and an acute medical issue arises, programs have been created to attempt to reduce unnecessary transitions to hospitals or emergency rooms. One such program is called INTERACT: Interventions to Reduce Acute Care Transfers (Pathway Health, 2021). The INTERACT program is designed for the medical staff members in long-term care centers to manage a resident's acute conditions and provides facilities with assessment and clinical diagnostic tools to reduce or eliminate a transfer where possible. The INTERACT program has been shown to improve self-reported pain in residents (Tappen et al., 2018) and decrease costs for both the resident and care communities (Ouslander et al., 2014). Sample strategies from the INTERACT program are highlighted in Exhibit 7.5.

Exhibit 7.5 Strategies to Avoid Unnecessary Resident Hospitalizations
- Implementing quality improvement processes with a dedicated team with a selected leader that also includes support from the care center administrator and the tracking of clearly defined measures and metrics for analysis.
- Evaluating any change to the resident's health at an early stage to manage their condition earlier and prevent unnecessary hospitalizations.
- Managing any changes to the resident's health that are more common and can be handled in the care center rather than the hospital.
- Increasing the use of advance directives or health care directives, as well as utilizing hospice or palliative care if selected by the resident.
- Enhancing the frequency and quality of communication between and among the facility administrator or executive director, staff members, family members, and hospitals, while documenting any communications.

Adapted from "The INTERACT Quality Improvement Program: An Overview for Medical Directors and Primary Care Clinicians in Long-Term Care" (Ouslander et al., 2014).

7.7   Essential Influencers

There are multiple clinicians and medical care providers in long-term care settings who play critical roles in ensuring residents are receiving the highest quality of care possible.

7.7.1   Medical Director and Director of Nursing

Two of the three members of the nursing home leadership triumvirate—the medical director and the director of nursing—are key members of care communities that can affect and improve the quality of care delivered to residents. If a resident has a primary care physician that is not the facility medical director, he or she must coordinate care with staff members in the care center to assure appropriate resident care that is modified when and where necessary to respond to any changes in the resident's health. The director of nursing in a care community plays an essential role to ensure other nursing staff are delivering care according to assessed needs and preferences and in alignment with the established care plan for each resident.

7.7.2 Nursing Staff and Nurse Aides

Beyond the director of nursing, the nursing staff and nurse aide staff members within the care community are essential contributors to a high quality of care. This includes the DON, RNs, licensed practical or vocational nurses (LPNs/LVNs), and CNAs. This group of individuals provides daily care, assists residents with their medications, and monitors residents across shifts in the care center to ensure continuity of care. The nurses and nurse aides may also assist residents after therapy sessions and observe residents to ensure their safety. In the United States, there are federal minimum staffing levels for RNs in nursing homes given the medical needs of nursing home residents, and some states require higher levels of nurse staffing depending on the acuity of residents in a given care center. Within assisted living centers serving higher acuity residents, nurses are often essential coordinators of any medical care provided. Although having RNs on staff may be ideal, especially for residents with cognitive impairment or who require assistance with medications, LPNs and LVNs still play a key role in coordinating care and assuring resident safety, even when the care provided is less complex.

7.7.3 Therapists and Service Staff

There are multiple therapy staff members employed by care centers or contracted to provide services within the building. Today, physical therapists, occupational therapists, speech-language pathologists, and therapy aides provide necessary rehabilitative care for residents and should be engaged during care planning processes to ensure appropriate goals are established, especially for residents who are able to return to their home following a shorter-term stay at the care community. In addition to therapy staff, housekeeping staff and dietary aides are also able to inform the care planning processes by reporting observations of resident behavior or other information gleaned from their relationships with residents, including preferences noted by residents, to better inform individualized care, which ultimately leads to enhanced quality of life.

References

Amirkhanyan, A. A., Kim, H. J., & Lambright, K. T. (2008). Does the public sector outperform the nonprofit and for-profit sectors? Evidence from a national panel study on nursing home quality and access. *Journal of Policy Analysis and Management, 27*(2), 326–353. https://doi.org/10.1002/pam.20327

Anderson, R. A., Hsieh, P. C., & Su, H. F. (1998). Resource allocation and resident outcomes in nursing homes: Comparisons between the best and worst. *Research in Nursing and Health,*

21(4), 297–313. https://doi.org/10.1002/(Sici)1098-240x(199808)21:4<297::Aid-Nur3>3.3. Co;2-F

Arling, G., Kane, R. L., Mueller, C., Bershadsky, J., & Degenholtz, H. B. (2007a). Nursing effort and quality of care for nursing home residents. *The Gerontologist, 47*(5), 672–682. https://doi.org/10.1093/geront/47.5.672

Arling, G., Lewis, T., Kane, R. L., Mueller, C., & Flood, S. (2007b). Improving quality assessment through multilevel modeling: The case of nursing home compare. *Health Services Research, 42*(3 Pt 1), 1177–1199. https://doi.org/10.1111/j.1475-6773.2006.00647.x

Castle, N. G. (2002). Nursing homes with persistent deficiency citations for physical restraint use. *Medical Care, 40*(10), 868–878. https://doi.org/10.1097/01.MLR.0000027357.74348.20

Castle, N. G. (2008). Nursing home caregiver staffing levels and quality of care: A literature review. *Journal of Applied Gerontology, 27*(4), 375–405. https://doi.org/10.1177/0733464808321596

Castle, N. G. (2011). Nursing home deficiency citations for abuse. *Journal of Applied Gerontology, 30*(6), 719–743. https://doi.org/10.1177/0733464811378262

Castle, N., Engberg, J., Lave, J., & Fischer, A. (2009). Factors associated with increasing nursing home closures. *Health Services Research, 44*(3), 1088–1109.

Castle, N. G., & Ferguson, J. C. (2010). What is nursing home quality and how is it measured? *The Gerontologist, 50*(4), 426–442. https://doi.org/10.1093/geront/gnq052

Centers for Medicare and Medicaid Services, United States Department of Health and Human Services. (2020, August). *Quality measures.* Retrieved from: https://www.cms.gov/Medicare/Quality-Initiatives-Patient-Assessment-Instruments/NursingHomeQualityInits/NHQIQualityMeasures.

Comondore, V. R., Devereaux, P. J., Zhou, Q., Stone, S. B., Busse, J. W., Ravindran, N. C., ... Guyatt, G. H. (2009). Quality of care in for-profit and not-for-profit nursing homes: Systematic review and meta-analysis. *British Medical Journal, 339*, 381–384. https://doi.org/10.1136/bmj.b2732

Davis, M. A. (1991). On nursing home quality: A review and analysis. *Medical Care Review, 48*(2), 129–166. https://doi.org/10.1177/002570879104800202

Degenholtz, H. B., Kane, R. A., Kane, R. L., Bershadsky, B., & Kling, K. C. (2006). Predicting nursing facility residents' quality of life using external indicators. *Health Services Research, 41*(2), 335–356. https://doi.org/10.1111/j.1475-6773.2005.00494.x

Dellefield, M. (2006). Interdisciplinary care planning and the written care plan in nursing homes: A critical review. *The Gerontologist, 46*(1), 128–133. https://doi.org/10.1093/geront/46.1.128

Donabedian, A. (1988). The quality of care: How can it be assessed? *JAMA, 260*(12), 1743–1748. https://doi.org/10.1001/jama.1988.03410120089033

Dove Healthcare Wissota Health and Regional Vent Center. (2021). *Ventilator and tracheostomy care.* Chippewa Falls, Wisconsin. Retrieved from https://www.dovehealthcare.com/ventilator_care.phtml.

Goergen, T. (2001). Stress, conflict, elder abuse and neglect in German nursing homes: A pilot study among professional caregivers. *Journal of Elder Abuse and Neglect, 13*(1), 1–26. https://doi.org/10.1300/J084v13n01_01

Good Samaritan Society – Specialty Care Community. (2021). *Huntington's disease care.* Robbinsdale, Minnesota. Retrieved from https://www.good-sam.com/services/long-term%20care/huntingtons-disease-care.

Grabowski, D. C., & Castle, N. G. (2004). Nursing homes with persistent high and low quality. *Medical Care Research and Review, 61*(1), 89–115. https://doi.org/10.1177/1077558703260122

Hansen, K. E., Hyer, K., Holup, A. A., Smith, K. M., & Small, B. J. (2019). Analyses of complaints, investigations of allegations, and deficiency citations in United States nursing homes. *Medical Care Research and Review, 76*(6), 736–757. https://doi.org/10.1177/1077558717744863

Harrington, C., Mullan, J. T., & Carrillo, H. (2004). State nursing home enforcement systems. *Journal of Health Politics, Policy and Law, 29*(1), 43–73. https://doi.org/10.1215/03616878-29-1-43

Hyer, K., Thomas, K. S., Branch, L. G., Harman, J. S., Johnson, C. E., & Weech-Maldonado, R. (2011). The influence of nurse staffing levels on quality of care in nursing homes. *Gerontologist, 51*(5), 610–616. https://doi.org/10.1093/geront/gnr050

Jogerst, G. J., Daly, J. M., Dawson, J. D., Peek-Asa, C., & Schmuch, G. (2006). Iowa nursing home characteristics associated with reported abuse. *Journal of the American Medical Directors Association, 7*(4), 203–207. https://doi.org/10.1016/j.jamda.2005.12.006

Johs-Artisensi, J. L. (2009). Promotion of best practices by regulatory agencies in nursing home closures and resident relocation. *Franklin Business and Law Journal, 4*, 94–109.

Johs-Artisensi, J. L., Hansen, K. E., & Olson, D. M. (2020). Qualitative analyses of nursing home residents' quality of life from multiple stakeholders' perspectives. *Quality of Life Research, 29*, 1229–1238. https://doi.org/10.1007/s11136-019-02395-3

Kaiser Family Foundation. (2015, May). *Reading the stars: Nursing home quality star ratings, nationally and by state.* Retrieved from: https://www.kff.org/medicare/issue-brief/reading-the-stars-nursing-home-quality-star-ratings-nationally-and-by-state/view/print/.

Kane, R. A. (2003). Definition, measurement, and correlates of quality of life in nursing homes: Toward a reasonable practice, research, and policy agenda. *The Gerontologist, 43*, 28–36. https://doi.org/10.1093/geront/43.suppl_2.28

Kane, R. L., Bershadsky, B., Kane, R. A., Degenholtz, H. H., Liu, J. J., Giles, K., & Kling, K. C. (2004). Using resident reports of quality of life to distinguish among nursing homes. *The Gerontologist, 44*(5), 624–632. https://doi.org/10.1093/geront/44.5.624

Kleinsorge, I. K., & Koenig, H. F. (1991). The silent customers: Measuring customer satisfaction in nursing homes. *Journal of Health Care Marketing, 11*(4), 2–13.

Landes, S. D., & Lillaney, N. (2019). Trend change in the intellectual disability nursing home census from 1977 to 2004. *American Journal on Intellecutal and Developmental Disabilities, 124*(5), 427–437. https://doi.org/10.1352/1944-7558-124.5.427

Lindbloom, E. J., Brandt, J., Hough, L. D., & Meadows, S. E. (2007). Elder mistreatment in the nursing home: A systematic review. *Journal of the American Medical Directors Association, 8*(9), 610–616. https://doi.org/10.1016/j.jamda.2007.09.001

Minnesota Department of Human Services. (2021). *Forensic services.* Saint Paul, Minnesota. Retrieved from https://mn.gov/dhs/people-we-serve/adults/services/forensic-services/.

Mor, V., Zinn, J., Angelelli, J., Teno, J. M., & Miller, S. C. (2004). Driven to tiers: Socioeconomic and racial disparities in the quality of nursing home care. *The Milbank Quarterly, 82*(2), 227–256. https://doi.org/10.1111/j.0887-378X.2004.00309.x

Naylor, M., & Keating, S. A. (2008). Transitional care: Moving patients from one care setting to another. *American Journal of Nursing, 108*(9 Suppl), 58–63. https://doi.org/10.1097/01.NAJ.0000336420.34946.3a

Netten, A., Darton, R., & Williams, J. (2003). Nursing home closures: Effects on capacity and reasons for closure. *Age and Ageing, 32*, 332–337.

Ouslander, J. G., Bonner, A., Herndon, L., & Shutes, J. (2014). The INTERACT quality improvement program: An overview for medical directors and primary care clinicians in long-term care. *Journal of the American Medical Directors Association, 15*(3), 162–170. https://doi.org/10.1016/j.jamda.2013.12.005

Pathway Health. (2021). *INTERACT: Lead with quality.* Lake Elmo, Minnesota. Retrieved from https://pathway-interact.com/.

Schofield, M. J., Powers, J. R., & Loxton, D. (2013). Mortality and disability outcomes of self-reported elder abuse: A 12-year prospective investigation. *Journal of the American Geriatrics Society, 61*(5), 679–685. https://doi.org/10.1111/jgs.12212

Shippee, T. P., Henning-Smith, C., Kane, R. L., & Lewis, T. (2013). Resident- and facility-level predictors of quality of life in long-term care. *The Gerontologist, 55*(4), 643–655. https://doi.org/10.1093/geront/gnt148

Spector, W. D., Selden, T. M., & Cohen, J. W. (1998). The impact of ownership type on nursing home outcomes. *Health Economics, 7*(7), 639–653. https://doi.org/10.1002/(SICI)1099-1050 (1998110)7:7<639::AID-HEC373>3.0.CO;2-0

Tappen, R. M., Newman, D., Huckfeldt, P., Yang, Z., Engstrom, G., Wolf, D. G., Shutes, J., Rojido, C., & Ouslander, J. G. (2018). Evaluation of nursing facility resident safety during implementation of the INTERACT quality improvement program. *Journal of the American Medical Directors Association, 19*(10), 907–913. https://doi.org/10.1016/j.jamda.2018.06.017

Teaster, P. B., Lawrence, S. A., & Cecil, K. A. (2007). Elder abuse and neglect. *Aging Health, 3*(1), 115–128. https://doi.org/10.1080/08946560903436130

Wayne County Nursing Home and Rehab Center. (2021). *Bariatric care.* Lyons, New York. Retrieved from https://waynecountynursinghome.org/bariatric-care.html

Chapter 8
Summary, Policy Recommendations, and Conclusions

Quality is everyone's responsibility. – W. Edwards Deming

Abstract Beyond the staff members in care centers—from the administrator, to the organization, to government-level agencies—there are practices and policies that can be created and aligned to support and enhance resident well-being. Organizational leadership strategies that administrators and executive directors can employ with residents, staff, and families are suggested in this chapter. Organizational support— whether in-house or at a broader corporate level—can also influence the culture and care delivered within individual care communities. Because of this, more macro-level policies and supports designed to focus on the resident, promote administrator independence, and enhance quality of life in care communities are discussed. Using existing research and currently implemented practices as a foundation, policy rec-ommendations incorporating governmental regulations and reimbursement method-ologies to enhance the resident experience are recommended. These proposed policy and leadership practice suggestions address and incorporate the various stakeholder groups, as applicable, and provide practical implementation strategies. Finally, conclusions are drawn which ultimately advocate for the enhanced planning and delivery of care and services in multiple long-term care settings to significantly improve quality of life for all residents.

Keywords Residents · Stakeholders · Resident-directed care · Family members · Champions · Chief influencers · Leadership · Person-centered care · Staffing · Onboarding · Continuing education · Resident satisfaction · Quality of life · Administrator role · Leadership team · Family communication · Organizational support · Reimbursement · Quality care · Policymaking · Regulation · Innovation · Staff satisfaction · Collaboration · Commitment

While the majority of this book has focused on the efforts and actions that care facilities and staff members therein can take to improve resident quality of life, it is important to remember that the primary, and most important, stakeholder of concern is the resident. The undercurrent in the prior chapters is the necessity to solicit resident input, assure residents' autonomy, and empower residents to direct their care and services however possible. In the most simplistic of ways, the resident is the "end user" that facilities must keep in mind and has the ability—more and more over time—to choose where they receive care and services, no matter their payment source. As noted in the introductory chapter, the global population is aging rapidly, with a large consumer base age 65 and older that is growing each year. This demographic shift has new and perhaps unexpected implications for congregate care centers and the customers (i.e., residents) they serve each day. Given this, as well as the increase in competition within and across services lines that promotes more resident choice, it is increasingly important to focus on improving resident satisfaction, and quality of life is one of the key drivers for this essential metric.

8.1 Care Recipients Should Direct their Care

In many countries, recently, the nomenclature and the approach within long-term care communities have shifted to "resident-centered," whereby decisions are made on the resident's behalf by others with the resident's best interests in mind. Any shift away from the institutionalized, medical model of care is ideal, because that alone tries to promote resident involvement and individualized care. While resident-centered care is well intentioned and, in practice, an approach that can yield beneficial outcomes for residents, this can leave open the very real possibility for paternalism to creep in. However and whenever possible, care and services should be *directed* by the resident, where the resident is an active, engaged member of the decision-making team and care and services are tailored to their specific needs, wants, and preferences. This can easily be accomplished through inclusion of the resident (and any persons the resident may wish to have present) in routine care conferences and care planning, as well as during the admissions process, where thorough inquiries and assessments of resident preferences and their life history can be ascertained to better tailor and individualize care.

When residents demonstrate cognitive impairment and cannot actively participate in decisions related to their care, then "resident-centered" presents as a more logical approach to pursue. In such cases, family members and friends of the individual may be wise sources of information to consult and include in decisions related to the resident, including those who may serve as a health care agent or be appointed by the court as a guardian for the person. In all of this, to note, some residents may indeed prefer to be less engaged in such decisions, which should also be respected and factored into decision-making in care centers.

8.2   Administrators as Champions and Chief Influencers

Administrators or executive directors of residential care communities have tremendous influence over the design, operations, and culture within the care center. The administrator is the ultimate leader who drives the culture of care and can ensure resident quality of life by building an organization that espouses the practices outlined in this book. Leaders must view resident needs comprehensively and holistically, prioritizing the principles of culture change by putting the resident at the center of their business model. With a strong philosophy of person-centered care underscoring an organization's mission, their leader can strategically empower caregivers to align and implement resident-driven practices, creating culture that maximizes residents' quality of life and emotional well-being.

The administrator is not alone in this; rather, they play a key role in setting the tone and leading by example. This includes hiring the right individuals to join their care team, in sufficient numbers and with the proper initial training required to deliver high-quality care to residents, and any specialized training that may be required for higher-needs populations served in the care center (e.g., residents who are ventilator dependent, residents with behavioral symptoms, residents with Huntington's disease). With staffing shortages in recent years, something significantly aggravated by the COVID-19 pandemic, some providers have resorted to hiring whomever they could find, regardless of that person's "fit" with the culture and mission of the care center. Other providers have turned to contract or pool staff from agencies to fill openings in staff or department schedules. Although this solves the immediate problem of filling a shift, such temporary staff members are not trained in the care philosophy and practices of the specific care center—and they are not instantly familiar with the particular preferences and needs of residents therein—which can negatively impact quality of care and quality of life in the long term.

While these approaches are indeed understandable during challenging times, ideally, administrators and executive directors would take great care in hiring staff members who demonstrate an ability to care for vulnerable residents and who are committed to a caring, respectful, resident-centered experience that promotes each of the domains discussed in this book. This does not have to be a drawn-out process, given recent evidence shows an importance to shorten the hiring process and get prospective staff members into training and earning wages more quickly, lest another industry (e.g., hotels, restaurants, retail stores) attract the person away. Beyond simply getting the new staff member hired, facility leadership needs to budget appropriate time to properly train the new employee and include training that ensures new staff members learn the culture and care philosophies of the facility, understand the importance of high-quality care, and develop skills to build relationships with residents and tailor care based on individual preferences. This training should both complement and supplement any required training for purposes of licensure or certification requirements in a given jurisdiction.

Beyond initial training and onboarding processes, care centers and leaders therein must ensure that staff members have the proper ongoing, continual education, tools, and support to meet residents' needs. With respect to ongoing education and training, programming should include routine reminders about how to foster community within the care center and deliver resident-driven care, adapted as necessary to the unique complement of residents. Administrators should also provide staff with practical and emotional support, and ensure they have the time, technology, and tools to deliver care effectively. Ongoing education necessarily must reinforce the multifaceted culture-based commitments of the facility to its residents and the surrounding community in efforts to assure quality of life and to aid in attracting both prospective staff and prospective residents. This requires a mental commitment, as well as a budgetary one, to set aside required funding for such programming. This ongoing education can help staff members maintain educational credits for licensure purposes, as well, but can be thoughtfully planned and structured to enhance the care delivery and resident experience at the same time. It should go without saying, but ongoing education needs to be tailored based on the unique needs of a facility's resident population and should be augmented or modified over time as that population may shift and change.

The administrator is ultimately responsible for assuring resident (as well as family and staff) satisfaction, which is a major component of quality of life. To accomplish this, an authentic culture of resident-centered care needs to be created, thoroughly implemented throughout all processes and facets of care delivery at the facility, and maintained over time. This includes orienting prospective residents and their family members to the care philosophy and practices during a prospective resident's tour of the care center; enshrining the culture and practices within the hiring process, onboarding, and initial training for all staff members; and continually assuring buy-in and commitment to culture during monthly events, meetings, and any ongoing training sessions. What leaders must understand is that one of the things staff most value about their roles is the ability to build relationships with residents, so a well-trained staff, encouraged to engage with residents to promote their psychosocial well-being, can reduce turnover and improve consistency of care for residents, which can and does lead to better quality care and quality of life.

Creating the infrastructure for these practices to flourish and championing a culture of broad community connections and resident well-being is the most important job of a care community's leader. There are several suggestions for the various staff members of care communities included in the prior domain-specific chapters, to align with quality of life practices that are important for resident satisfaction. The administrator role is discussed here as the leadership position that must cohesively bring everyone together and lead in a way that promotes engagement by all staff members into the desired culture. This includes establishing and routinely working with a leadership team within the building, comprised of the various department heads (e.g., director of nursing, maintenance director), to ensure all these community leaders and managers view their own roles as creators of a culture of resident-centered care, developing their department staff in the organizations' philosophy of care, and focus on ensuring staff satisfaction, as well. When the leadership team prioritizes and takes care of the care center's staff members, they too in turn will take care of residents and ensure a high-quality experience all throughout the building.

Although the administrator's primary responsibilities are to create and maintain the tone of the organizational culture and ensure smooth business operations through their management of policies, procedures, and personnel, another important role within that is ensuring healthy communications with both residents and family members. If administrators truly embrace a resident-centered philosophy, they must make getting to know their care recipients a priority. One easy strategy for this is by conducting "daily rounds"—this gives the administrator an opportunity to walk through the care community—using all their senses, to observe the physical environment as well as the activities and engagement of residents, staff, and any visitors. Greeting residents by name, stopping for periodic conversations with people, and lending a helping hand, on occasion, is a beneficial way to better get to know individuals and to demonstrate the administrator's commitment to prioritizing residents as well as their connectedness to the care community. While communications with residents may be somewhat easier to facilitate, since they live where the administrator works, communication with and successful engagement of families can be more challenging. Several strategies for facilitating family communication and engagement have been emphasized throughout this book, especially in the chapters related to relationships and activities. Not only does the administrator have to figure out *that* they need to communicate with families, they also must take into consideration how best to deliver a message that families will hear and absorb. For example, even if an administrator's preferred way of communicating is through emails or newsletters, families' preferences may differ. Never was the need for administrators to communicate effectively with families greater than during the recent COVID-19 pandemic and, luckily, several creative, engaging communication strategies have been borne from this difficult event. An important lesson learned is that one-way communication may no longer be enough, and that families may expect two-way communication (i.e., receiving input from family members through social media posts or via family council meetings) which may benefit all parties. Now that many care facilities are equipped with the technology to use video conferencing to involve families in resident care planning or to conduct interactive monthly or bimonthly briefings, where families can obtain organization updates and people can ask questions and receive answers in real time, these are tools that should continue to be used. Some countries have regulations that may require administrators to allow the establishment of family councils within their buildings, but to best support care recipients' quality of life, all administrators should be encouraging such councils to form, as families possess a wealth of knowledge that is beneficial to supporting and advancing resident well-being throughout the entire care community. Beyond the internal benefit of listening to families and incorporating them into the care provided to residents, their increased satisfaction with care for their loved one has been shown to create positive public ambassadors in the surrounding community and may generate future referrals through word-of-mouth marketing.

8.3   Organizational and Leadership Support

For long-term care organizations to successfully provide care, such that residents' quality of life and emotional well-being are supported and uplifted, a certain amount of financial resources are needed. Obviously, if resources were unlimited, so too would be opportunities to build beautiful, brand new care campuses, equip them with the latest technology, and hire an excess of abundantly qualified staff. However, the reality for most long-term care providers is they are operating on relatively tight budgets and thin profit margins. In countries where government resources are used to fund long-term care, ensuring that government reimbursement rates are adequate to meet both the basic health care and critical psychosocial needs of residents will best support providers in delivering care that increases resident quality of life.

Beyond financial resources to provide excellent care to residents, there is also evidence to suggest the importance of companies hiring the right administrators or executive directors for the care centers within the organization. Once companies have great leaders in place, trust and autonomy in the administrator to allow him or her to direct the practices within their building is of utmost importance. With corporate office support, including regional directors supporting newer administrators as they begin in a care center and back office support for financials and effective billing practices, and independence to act, administrators have the ability to tailor practices to best suit resident preferences and needs (e.g., managing staff schedules to optimize care), implement an individualized management style, structure the physical environment and service lines to meet strategic objectives, or create a presence with local organizations and community members. Autonomous administrators can also enhance the resident experience and cater care and services to attract prospective residents, keeping the beds in the building as full as possible by utilizing innovative practices with surrounding community partners. Additionally, with such independence, the administrator can work collaboratively with the resident council and family council to truly individualize care for the facility's residents. This not only improves quality of life, but has the additional benefit of creating a more positive public persona for the care center, engendering surrounding community members to be incorporated into activities and events for the residents, and also potentially motivating community members to consider the facility for their own future long-term care needs.

Finally, to ensure the best quality of life and quality care is experienced by all residents, at the facility level, the bulk of all excess revenues generated beyond covering expenses should be thoughtfully reinvested back into staffing (e.g., adequate wages and benefits, appropriate resident-staff ratios), food, activities and events, equipment and technology, caregiver training, community engagement, building remodeling, and innovative quality improvement initiatives. Likely, these investments will show great return in the form of happier residents, families, and staff, as well as enhanced organizational stability, higher census, and revenue growth.

8.4 Opportunities for Government Licensure and Regulatory Agencies

On the more macro level, beyond what can be done within individual care communities or even at the organizational or corporate level, the laws, regulations, and policies set by governmental authorities must be carefully constructed and routinely evaluated. In policymaking, evaluating the actual effect of new (or revised) policies, to assure that intent matches the obtained outcomes, often goes unaccomplished or takes many years to occur. Some policies specific to facilities serving older adults may constrict the ability of administrators, executive directors, and their staff to customize care and services to delight customers and exceed resident expectations. What may begin as intended policy to protect residents and provide a minimum level of care or safety ultimately may inhibit potential approaches that residents themselves may request or would permit facilities to attract new residents based on assessment of market demands in a given geographic area. That said, there should be standards which codify a minimum threshold of resident quality of life for care centers. For example, in the United States, there are several regulations and standards which must be implemented to ensure an appropriate quality of life for residents, with penalties assessed to providers for any noncompliance. This includes the right to participate in planning one's care, have one's needs and preferences incorporated (i.e., tailoring care to the individual), self-determination (i.e., autonomy), having a safe and homelike environment, and activities that meet the interests and preferences of individual care recipients.

Ideally, government entities could and should implement more effective ways for care communities to pilot new and innovative methods of delivering care and services for residents, based on their unique needs and wants. Too often, at least in the United States, administrators and staff may be apprehensive about attempting a revamped process tailored to residents out of fear of regulatory citations and accompanying fines and fees. This chilling effect was likely not intended when the regulations designed to protect residents were implemented but, nonetheless, such is the effect that has evolved over time. Government authorities might engage with care communities more proactively by enabling waiver programs to allow new programs and processes to be tested without apprehension over impending sanctions. Such a process could lead to better customization of facility practices to enhance quality of life and, indeed, quality of care. Additionally, government agencies must weigh the necessary criteria to certify or license a staff member against the need to give providers and administrators requisite flexibility to accelerate the hiring process—appropriately—with the staffing shortages that are inherent in the long-term care industry. With too many unnecessary regulatory hurdles and barriers, care centers face the very real risk of losing talented staff members to other industries due to a delay in getting started because of onerous licensure or certification requirements.

Many of the suggestions and noted best practices in prior chapters could be implemented right now, with no changes to legal or regulatory standards if care communities simply took the initiative to modify their current practices. However, increased flexibility to allow facilities to augment existing practices—within specified parameters and assuring a safe environment of care—without fear of reprisal could incentivize innovations and individualization that truly create a homelike environment and grants residents autonomy to have more input into care practices and service offerings. The tendency is often to craft laws or regulations which are predicated on easily identifiable and measurable metrics, which are more quantitative in nature and more applicable to the quality of care delivered. However, when prioritizing and working to enhance quality of life, the meaningful impacts of such efforts may be better assessed subjectively and qualitatively—and are, admittedly, more difficult to measure. However, customer satisfaction surveys, including whether residents or families might recommend a care center to other prospective residents (e.g., net promoter scores), are currently used in acute care and long-term care settings and could be utilized to drive reimbursement and funding to those sites which prioritize resident satisfaction and strive to improve quality of life.

In addition, regulatory structures and resources could be more thoughtfully used to support quality improvement. For example, in the United States, when facilities are cited for operating outside of strict compliance with regulations, they are often required to pay significant fines. One suggestion is that governments could put financial resources accumulated through these fines to specific good use to improve quality for residents. Perhaps these monies could be used to develop "strike teams" of experts, armed with best practices to rapidly assist in quality improvements, rather than waiting for already struggling organizations to figure out solutions on their own. Another suggestion might be to quickly and easily return those dollars back to targeted long-term care communities that have a history of poor quality or lack of resources—marketing the availability of these funds and a simple process to make appropriate awards to facilities with outcome-based projects designed to improve resident care and quality of life. This could include funding the building of outdoor garden spaces, resources to support integrated resident-family events, more modern or specialized therapeutic equipment, or purchasing technology to enhance resident autonomy.

A lack of financial resources and staffing challenges in long-term care, which can make it more difficult to implement practices that enhance quality of life, are not unique to the United States. Many countries with universal health care systems covering the populous and that include support for long-term care experience similar challenges. If the intent of countries who regulate and, either in part or in full, offer reimbursement for long-term services and supports, stems from a desire to protect societies' most vulnerable individuals, then in the context of person-centered care such "protection" is redefined as maximizing residents' quality of life. Government regulations and reimbursement structures should be designed to support providers in meeting both residents' physical and psychosocial needs, and facilities' success in protecting older adults will be evident in enhanced quality of life metrics.

8.5   The Imperative and Charge to Improve Resident Quality of Life

When in proper alignment, facility practices, governmental laws and regulations, and appropriate allocation of public and private resources can truly support innovative practices and strategies that individualize care and services for residents. Such coordination can truly serve to improve the overall quality of care and services, while also assuring a quality, homelike environment. In many cases, it is truly up to the administrator or executive director to establish a culture that prioritizes residents, tailors care and services to resident preferences, and empowers staff to continually improve quality of life in buildings. However, policies implemented through governmental laws and regulations, as well as the funding and reimbursement mechanisms established to provide care, must not hinder the ability of leaders and their staff members to maximize resident quality of life.

While the vast majority of research and practices discussed in this book focus on residents, it cannot be understated that these suggested practices have significant effects on staff members, too. Research has indicated time and again that when staff feel supported, happy, and able to provide care tailored to residents, the residents themselves are happier and report a higher quality of life. And when residents are satisfied, most often there is a reciprocal effect on staff—and so goes this cycle in care centers with elated, happy residents. Many of the care centers that observe both high resident satisfaction and high staff satisfaction have implemented cultures that are homelike, promote resident respect and autonomy, enable staff to develop meaningful relationships with those for whom they care, and appropriately tailor care and services to exceed what residents may even expect.

Not every practice discussed in this book requires substantial financial investment. Having a pleasant demeanor, developing a resident-directed or even a resident-centered culture, assessing residents' needs and preferences, and tailoring care and services to please residents, as examples, can be easily implemented to promote a high level of quality of life in care centers that exist today, without further investment of resources. The domain-specific chapters in this book intentionally highlight practices already in effect many places, in an effort to show what is indeed in the realm of possible under current regulations and reimbursement practices.

While collaboration and commitment are key to continually improving resident well-being and satisfaction, a comprehensive culture of quality of life and autonomy must permeate throughout the care community. While sufficient evidence and rationale have been provided throughout this book to enhance resident quality of life, consumers are increasingly demanding such practices, making it even more important to respect, prioritize, and incorporate resident-focused care and services in their new home. The strategies provided in this book are merely a starting point for various stakeholders, but with thoughtful involvement of residents in individual care communities, the blueprint evolves for augmenting resident satisfaction and quality of life that will transform care and excite current and prospective residents. If older adult residents are truly valued, then it is a moral imperative that words and actions align to assure efforts aimed at promoting quality of care and quality of life are attempted, sustained, and successful.

Appendix

Prior to selecting a new home for oneself or a loved one, when increased supports and services are needed, ideally one should have an opportunity to meet with leadership and caregiver representatives of the prospective care community (e.g., the administrator or executive director, an admissions coordinator, and even direct caregivers) and take a tour. While touring the care community, the prospective resident or family members should take the opportunity to both observe the surroundings, activities, and "feeling" of the culture, and should also interact, converse, and ask questions, as they are able, of leadership, caregivers, and even current care recipients or their family members—including asking questions of residents who may have a form of dementia or other cognitive impairment. Making a decision to move to a new "home" is a big one, so it is important to take the time to visit— perhaps on multiple occasions, and at different times of the day—to be sure that everyone involved in the decision-making process has enough information to feel comfortable and confident that they or their loved one will have good quality of life in their new home.

What follows is a checklist of questions, built specifically around the six major quality of life domains discussed in this book, as well as the practices therein. There are numerous factors that likely go into a decision about which care community is ultimately the best fit for you or a loved one, and if quality of life and well-being matters to you or to them, this is information worth exploring. While there are several items to inquire about or observe under each domain, below, you should select the items of importance to you when touring or visiting a prospective care community. There are many other tools and resources available from various organizations that may be used to facilitate decisions about when the time is right and what the best setting may be to meet an individual's or a loved one's needs, and a sample of such resources can be found at the end of this appendix.

Checklist of Questions and Observations to Consider When Assessing Quality of Life Factors Prior to Selecting a New Long-Term Care Community

© The Author(s), under exclusive license to Springer Nature Switzerland AG 2022
J. L. Johs-Artisensi, K. E. Hansen, *Quality of Life and Well-Being for Residents in Long-Term Care Communities*, Human Well-Being Research and Policy Making, https://doi.org/10.1007/978-3-031-04695-7

Autonomy, Respect, Dignity, and Sense of Purpose

• Questions for Provider—Administration and Staff Members

Do you have a person-centered care philosophy?

What is the resident-staff ratio?

How much turnover in administrative and caregiver staff has there been in the past year?

Are your staff trained in person-centered care principles?

Are staff trained in hospitality principles?

Do residents have a say in their daily schedule?

Are residents able to get up and go to bed when they wish?

Are residents' bathing preferences (e.g., bath or shower, time of day) honored?

Are residents (and their families) able to participate in their own care planning process?

What educational opportunities are there for residents to learn new things?

Do you have a resident council? How active are the members in the council?

• Other Observations

Do you see caregivers treating residents with respect?

Are residents smiling?

Are caregivers smiling?

Are residents engaged in activities?

• Questions for Current Care Recipients

Do you enjoy living here?

Do you feel like you have a sense of purpose here?

Do you feel like you belong to the community here?

Do you feel that the caregivers respect your privacy?

Do you feel like staff have taken the time to get to know you as a person?

Relationships

• Questions for Provider—Administration and Staff Members

How do you help residents, with common interests, connect with each other?

How do you support residents who have become friends if one moves to another part of the building/campus?

How do you assist residents in staying connected with their peers if they are required to spend time in isolation or quarantine?

What opportunities for meaningful interactions do residents have here?

Do you use consistent staffing assignments?

Do the staff receive training in "soft skills" like customer service, hospitality, and how to facilitate relationships?

Do you have a staff-resident "buddy" program?

Do you have a peer ambassador, welcome committee, or greeter program—either formal or informal?

How do you support residents through the grieving process when other residents pass away?

Are staff encouraged to spend time developing personal relationships with residents?

Are nurse aides involved in the resident care planning process?

Are staff's interests in developing relationships with residents considered as part of the hiring process?

What part about working here you enjoy the most?

How are caregivers supported when residents pass away?

(continued)

Are family visits encouraged, even if modifications are in place during periods of isolation or quarantine?

Are there specific visiting hours? Can visitors come anytime? Can family stay overnight on occasion?

Is there technology assistance for helping residents have video visits with family?

How are family members able to participate in the resident care planning process? Are they scheduled at convenient or flexible times for working family members? Is teleconferencing or videoconferencing an option?

Are staff able to support residents in going on off-site outings, like to a store or a restaurant?

Are residents able to leave the care center to make visits home to visit family or pets? What process is there for doing so? Can they be gone overnight?

Are families allowed to help their loved one with activities of daily living or other care tasks at the care center?

Do you have an active family council? How often do they meet and when? How have you addressed their concerns or suggestions for changes related to residents in the care center?

Do you have a resident/family orientation program or handbook?

What type of family engagement activities does the care center typically sponsor (e.g., a spring carnival, special holiday dinners)?

How do you regularly communicate with families (e.g., newsletters, social media, webinar briefings)?

Are there any family support groups or educational seminars offered?

How do you prefer families communicate with administration (e.g., email, open door policy, suggestion box)?

What processes are in place for handling any resident or family member complaints?

Are romantic relationships between residents supported?

Do you have a sexual expression policy?

Is there an "intimacy room" or other private space option for those with shared room arrangements?

Do you have a social worker in your care center who is skilled in facilitating resident relationships?

Do you have an activities director who values family engagement?

Are residents regularly, personally invited to join in activities that align with their interests?

Is there an active volunteer program?

Do the staff or caregivers speak the language of the prospective resident?

• Observations

Do you see residents socializing with each other?

Are the interactions you see between caregivers and residents warm, polite, and respectful?

Do you notice residents socializing with each other or engaging in activities with each other, outside of formal activities programs?

Is the dining room set up to encourage conversation and relationship building? And are residents encouraged to leave their rooms for meals and socialization?

Do you see care recipients having conversations with tablemates in the dining room during meals?

Do you hear laughter within the care community?

Do staff have easy-to-read name badges? Do their badges include pictures, especially if masks are being worn?

(continued)

Do you see caregivers addressing residents by name?

Do residents appear to be clean and well groomed?

Do you see caregivers talking with residents as they transport them or otherwise assist them?

• Questions for Current Care Recipients

Do you think of some of your caregivers as friends or family?

Are the caregivers good listeners? Do they talk to you while they are helping you?

Do staff knock before they enter your room? Do they maintain your privacy as much as possible when caring for you?

Do caregivers call you by your preferred name?

Activities and Religion

• Questions for Provider—Administration and Staff Members

Are there an assortment of activities planned each day or each week to give residents variety?

Can residents choose to take part in the activities they wish to, including if residents are unable to leave their room or have mobility issues?

Do the activities scheduled promote safe, physical activity? Do the activities promote cognitive stimulation and engagement?

Do you involve the therapy department with scheduling activities to assure activities with a physical component are also safe?

Do the residents get to help plan the activities offered in the care center?

Does the care center offer the religious or cultural support that residents might need? What arrangements are made to meet resident needs, if not?

Does your care center use any technology within your activities (e.g., gaming systems, computers, tablets, virtual reality headsets)?

What types of activities do you schedule that are mentally stimulating to help challenge residents with dementia or cognitive impairments?

Are there activities scheduled outdoors in safe spaces around the care center? Are there activities scheduled in the community where residents can travel outside of the care center?

How do you provide activities for residents with dementia or cognitive impairment? Do you utilize activity stations for residents with dementia?

Are volunteers recruited and used within the care center to facilitate smaller group activities or more one-on-one activities with residents?

How many residents normally participate in the activities scheduled?

What do staff members do to encourage isolated residents to participate in activities?

What cultural events are scheduled throughout the year to respond to the preferences or beliefs of your residents?

Do you have a chapel or other dedicated space for religious or spiritual services?

Is there a clergy member or faith leader on staff to lead religious services or faith-based activities (e.g., bible study)? Do you have arrangements with other faith leaders in the community to be available, as needed, for residents?

How do you try to incorporate family members into the activities or special events at this care center?

Do you do any special events for residents who might be veterans (e.g., Memorial Day or Veterans day celebrations)?

• Observations

Do you see residents engaging in activities with staff members and/or fellow residents?

(continued)

Are there any activity stations placed throughout the care center for residents with dementia?

In common areas in the care center, do you notice any books, games, or other materials set out for residents to engage in activities and socialization?

Ask for a copy of the activities schedule for the week or the month. Do you see activities scheduled throughout each day? Are there activities planned during the weekends rather than just during the week?

Does the care center have a variety of spaces available for activities—including larger spaces for groups and smaller spaces for more solitary activities—throughout the building or campus?

• Questions for Current Care Recipients

Do you feel there are a good variety of activities here for you to participate in?

Do you have the choice to participate in the activities you find appealing?

Do you have the option to do something more solitary when preferred rather than group activities?

Are you satisfied with the care center staff in how they listen to your ideas for any activities?

Do you feel that you have a good variety of activities to participate in even during periods of isolation or quarantine?

Environment

• Questions for Provider—Administration and Staff Members

Is a "household" model being used?

How many people live on each household/ neighborhood/unit/floor and how many total are in the care community?

Are furniture and technology supplied for short-term residents?

Are long-term residents allowed to bring their own furniture?

Are private rooms available?

If a shared room is required, are residents able to choose their own roommate?

Are residents allowed to have or supplied with a mini-refrigerator for their personal room?

Do residents have an option to keep any possessions in their rooms in locked cabinets or drawers?

Are residents allowed to hang pictures on the walls?

Are residents allowed to paint their walls or select the paint color?

Are families encouraged to help residents to move in, decorate, and get settled in?

Are maintenance personnel available to assist with moving furniture or hanging items on walls?

Are residents allowed to personalize or decorate their exterior doors or hallway space outside their bedrooms?

Can residents control the temperature of their personal rooms?

If rooms are shared, are wireless headphones available for television or radio listening?

Is wifi available in resident rooms? In common areas? What about cable television?

Are residents allowed to use technology assistants (e.g., Amazon Alexa) in their rooms?

Can you explain the bathing process and whether bathing occurs on a schedule?

Are telephones available in resident rooms or only in common spaces?

Is there a daycare onsite or partnerships with schools that would bring children into the care community?

(continued)

Do residents have access or opportunity to be involved in cooking in a residential kitchen?

Are safe spaces available to support residents who wander?

What environmental cues are used to assist residents with orientation and wayfinding?

Hope do you prevent elopement of residents with dementia?

Have you received any citations on your last annual survey related to environmental hazards or the safety of residents (e.g., Life Safety Code)? How did you correct these issues?

• Observations

Does the care community feel homelike?

Is it free of undesirable odors?

Does the environment look clean and in good repair?

Are any elements of "outside" brought indoors (e.g., exterior architecture, nature/ greenery)?

Are the personal rooms adequately sized?

Is there ample seating, storage, and work space in your personal room for the way you hope to use the space?

Are there shelves or other spaces to display photographs and your other personal belongings?

Will you have adequate space to engage in leisure time in your personal room (e.g., a desk to write at or do puzzles, space for a computer or CD player, a comfortable chair to sit in)?

If a shared room is necessary, are there ways to preserve privacy for each of you (e.g., a partial wall, an ample privacy curtain)?

If a shared room is necessary, can each person see out the window? Can each person get to their own bed or to the bathroom without intruding on the other's space?

Is there an attached bathroom with a shower? Is it equipped with safety equipment (e.g., grab bars, hand rails)?

Are residents' rooms decorated in their own personal style?

Do the different neighborhoods, units, or floors have unique names?

What do any shared bathing spaces (e.g., spas, shower rooms) look like?

Is a whirlpool tub available?

Are personalized bathing products or aromatherapy scents incorporated into bathing?

Are mirrors installed on a tilt so residents in wheelchairs can see their reflections from a seated position?

Are there any warming elements in the spa or tub room (e.g., towel warmers, heated lamps, heated floors)?

Are seating areas welcoming and comfortable looking?

Are residents using common spaces for visiting or their own enjoyment (e.g., playing cards, doing puzzles, knitting, reading)?

Are common areas decorated with tasteful décor or pictures of the people who live there?

Is the furniture in common spaces comfortable? Is seating arranged to encourage socializing and engaging in activities with each other?

Are spaces available where you could host a small group of guests with some privacy?

Are the types of common spaces you would enjoy available (e.g., television lounge, library, movie theater, game room, beauty shop, chapel, bistro, fitness center, residential laundry room, gift shop)?

Do you see caregivers at workspaces that are located near common areas and are accessible to all residents?

(continued)

Are the activity spaces separate from the dining room?

Do you see any pets living in the care community?

Do you see resident-accessible bathrooms near common spaces, like lounges or the dining room?

Do doorways and hallways seem easy to navigate (e.g., wide enough, free of clutter, handrails)?

Are there smaller, decentralized dining room options available?

Do dining rooms feel either homelike or restaurant-like in nature?

During meal times is the dining room distractingly noisy?

Is the smell of appetizing food present in the building?

Are paint colors pretty and pleasing to the eye?

Is there adequate lighting indoors, including plenty of natural light?

Do you hear alarms, overhead pages, or an abundance of other annoying ambient noises?

Is the temperature in common areas comfortable?

Are there plenty of opportunities to observe interesting outdoor views from inside?

Are there safe, attractive, and functional outdoor spaces available to residents?

Are outdoor spaces equipped with safety features like smooth walking pathways, handrails, seating, and shade?

Are outdoor spaces equipped with tools and equipment to engage in activities (e.g., gardening tools, lawn games)?

• Questions for Current Care Recipients

Do you feel comfortable here?

Are you able to get the support to use the available spaces the way you would like to (e.g., Beauty shop, garden spaces, library)?

How often are you able to go outside?

How often are you able to leave the facility on a community outing?

Food

• Questions for Provider—Administration and Staff Members

Do residents have a choice of food items from the menu at each meal?

Can each resident decide when he or she would like to eat? Is there a regimented schedule that residents must follow?

Do residents have a choice of where they'd like to eat? If eating in a dining area, do residents have some choice in who their tablemates are?

If the residents have special dietary needs (e.g., low-salt, no-sugar-added), can you provide that?

How do you assess residents to know whether they need modified foods (e.g., pureed, liquified) or thickened liquids to have proper hydration and nutrition?

If residents are unable or unwilling to consume "normal" foods, what's your policy and approach for using supplements to provide appropriate nutrition?

Do you have "normal" foods available for residents (e.g., mashed potatoes, yogurt, pudding) if they do not wish to have a pureed meal?

If needed, are there staff members available to help residents eat and drink at meal times?

Are there nutritious snacks available for residents throughout the day? How do residents "order" those when hungry or thirsty?

(continued)

How do you assess residents' satisfaction with food? How do you assess the family members' satisfaction with food?

How often is your dietician on duty in the care center? Is your dietician routinely included during care planning processes to assure proper hydration and nutrition for residents in the care center?

For residents with any swallowing disorders (e.g., dysphagia), how do the nursing staff and medical director assess such issues and work with the dietician to modify the presentation of food or liquids?

If any residents are underweight or dehydrated, how do you respond to help the resident return to a healthy state of nutrition or hydration?

During meals, how do you help promote socialization among residents to ensure an enjoyable dining experience that promotes healthy eating behaviors?

Have you received any citations related to food storage, food preparation, or food service to residents? If so, how have you corrected those deficiencies to make sure food is safe for residents to consume?

During meal times, what do you do to enhance the ambiance to make the dining experience enjoyable? Do you play music? Do you set out seasonal table decorations or holiday decorations during certain times of the year?

Can you explain how you involve residents in the planning of meals and menus? Do you have a resident advisory committee that works with your food services director?

Do you have any nontraditional sources of food (e.g., garden at the care center where residents can grow vegetables that are incorporated into meals)?

Do you try to have a restaurant-style or homelike-style dining environment? What is the terminology used to refer to staff members assisting during meals (e.g., feeding assistant, server, waiter/waitress)?

Are staff members allowed to eat meals with residents to have enhanced socialization (including having a meal when not assisting a resident with eating or drinking)?

Are the plates, silverware, table mats or tablecloths, and decorations planned with colors that enhance the dining experience for residents with dementia or residents with visual impairments?

• Observations

Is it easy to navigate from the hallway area to a specific table in the dining area?

When residents are eating, are they using facility-like plastic cups, plastic silverware, and paper napkins? Or are they using cups, plates, metal silverware, and cloth napkins that are more homelike?

Do you hear any music playing or notice any environmental decoration that improves the dining area and looks more homelike?

Do residents appear to be having conversations with their tablemates? Do residents appear to be socializing or having conversations with staff members nearby?

Is food being served to residents on plates? Or is food served using a more cafeteria-style tray?

Is food cooked and served on the unit or in the specific dining area? Or is food rolled out using more industrial-style food carts (i.e., warming carts)?

Are there any snacks set out for residents to have between meals? Are there any "cafés" where residents can order a snack between meals?

• Questions for Current Care Recipients

How would you rate the quality of the food in the care center?

(continued)

Do you feel you have some choice in what food you eat at each meal?

Do you think there is enough variety in the meals served here?

How would you rate the portion size of meals here? Do you get enough to eat?

Do you think there are adequate snacks available between meals?

How would you rate the dining atmosphere during meals?

Do you enjoy your tablemates and your ability to socialize during meals?

What would you change about the menus or food served in this care center if you could?

Quality of Care

• Questions for Provider—Administration and Staff Members

What is the current quality rating of this care center (e.g., CMS 5-Star Rating)? What are your ratings for surveys/inspections, quality measures, and staffing?

Are you a for profit or nonprofit care center?

What percentage of your residents are short-stay residents (e.g., receiving therapy for recuperation following a hospital stay) and what percentage are long-stay?

How many citations were received on your last annual survey related to quality measures for resident care? How have you corrected any of those deficiencies?

How many complaints were made in the prior year to surveyors? How many of those resulted in a citation to this care center?

Have you been required to pay any fines if you have received citations (e.g., civil monetary penalties)?

What is your process for resolving a complaint within the care center before a resident would contact the state agency or ombudsman?

If a resident has their own doctor, how do you arrange for the resident to see that physician rather than the care center's medical director? If there is a personal physician, how does he or she coordinate with the nursing staff in the care center?

In case of any emergency, does this care center have a relationship with a nearby hospital? If so, which hospital? Can residents (or family members) choose to go to a different hospital if they wish to?

Do you and your staff leadership team check to ensure you don't hire any staff members with a finding of abuse, neglect, or financial exploitation? Or that you don't hire any staff members who are prevented from providing care because of prior maltreatment?

How would I or my loved one report concerns about the care and safety of residents?

What initial training is provided to staff members to ensure they are properly trained to provide appropriate care for residents? What type(s) of ongoing training do you provide to assure staff members stay up-to-date with best practices of providing care?

Is there an appropriate number of licensed nursing staff on duty, based on the acuity of residents in the care center?

How many direct care staff members (e.g., nurse aides, RNs) are available to help residents during the day, at night, and on weekends?

How do you assure that you have appropriately trained staff providing care and services to residents in this care center?

Are any of your staff cross-trained to provide various care and services (e.g., nurse aides trained to assist residents at meal times)?

If a resident has dementia or other cognitive impairment, what care practices are employed before medication is used (e.g., behavioral interventions before an antipsychotic, antidepressant, or antianxiety medication is given)?

(continued)

What types of memory care are provided to residents who may have mild cognitive impairment, behavioral issues from dementia, or more pronounced cognitive or physical impairments because of dementia?

How are care plans updated in this care center? How do residents or family members raise a concern if they note a change in condition?

If you admit a resident from a hospital, how do you coordinate with the hospital staff members to assure a smooth transition? Which staff members are in charge of coordinating with hospital staff and following up with residents once admitted to the care center?

• Observations

Do you notice any residents "parked" at the nursing station that are not being engaged with in some way?

Are there any call lights that stay on for an unusually long period of time while you are visiting the care center?

Ask to see their therapy space, where physical therapy, occupational therapy, or speech-language therapy is provided. Does their equipment appear to be in good repair? Do they have a variety of devices or "stations" to assist residents who need therapy?

During your visit to the care center, do you notice staff members walking about and interacting with residents? Do you see staff members clustering in areas that residents don't have access to?

• Questions for Current Care Recipients

Do you feel like you are getting good quality medical care and services in this care center?

Do you think the nurse aides like their jobs?

Do you think the nurses (i.e., RNs, LPN/LVNs) like their jobs?

Do you feel like the staff members honestly try to provide care and services that align with your personal preferences and wishes?

Do you know who your doctor is (i.e., medical director of the care center, personal physician outside the care center)? Do you think your doctor listens to your concerns and incorporates your preferences into the care you receive?

Do you feel like staff members interact honestly with you? Do you trust the staff members when they tell you something?

Do you feel the therapists (e.g., physical therapy, occupational therapy, speech-language therapy) listen to you and are helping you during sessions? Do you feel like the therapists coordinate well with the nursing staff and medical director to manage your pain appropriately?

Do you feel that you get enough time in therapy?

Are there any issues that have been raised by the resident council or family council that you feel have not been adequately addressed by leaders in this care community?

Sample Resources to Support Care Recipients and Families in the Care Decision-Making Process

• Pioneer Network:

   https://www.pioneernetwork.net/elders-families/questions-to-ask/

• The National Consumer Voice for Quality Long-Term Care:

   https://theconsumervoice.org/news/detail/news_list/advocating-for-quality-nurs
      ing-home-care-help

- Medicare.gov Nursing Home Checklist:

    https://www.medicare.gov/care-compare/en/assets/resources/nursing-home/
    NursingHomeChecklist_Oct_2019.pdf

- Medicare.gov Care Compare Website:

    https://www.medicare.gov/care-compare/

- Alzheimer's Association:

    https://www.alzheimers.net/2014-04-24-questions-to-ask-about-memory-care

- A Place for Mom:

    https://www.aplaceformom.com/assisted-living

- AARP Tips on Finding a Nursing Home:

    https://www.aarp.org/caregiving/basics/info-2019/finding-a-nursing-home.html

Printed in Great Britain
by Amazon

49449021R00130